Rare Kidney Tumors

Gabriel G. Malouf • Nizar M. Tannir
Editors

Rare Kidney Tumors

Comprehensive Multidisciplinary Management and Emerging Therapies

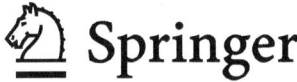 Springer

Editors
Gabriel G. Malouf
Department of Hematology and Oncology
Strasbourg University Hospital
Hopital Civil
Strasbourg
France

Nizar M. Tannir
Department of Genitourinary
Medical Oncology
MD Anderson Cancer Center
Houston, Texas
USA

ISBN 978-3-030-07281-0   ISBN 978-3-319-96989-3   (eBook)
https://doi.org/10.1007/978-3-319-96989-3

This Springer imprint is published by the registered company Springer Nature Switzerland AG
The registered company address is: Gewerbestrasse 11, 6330 Cham, Switzerland

Tannir's Dedication:
"I would like to dedicate this book to my wife Nada and our three children, Zane, Ryan, and Jana, for their love and support; to my mentees and colleagues, Gaby Malouf and Pavlos Msaouel, for enriching my life with their friendship, and for their important contributions to the field of rare kidney tumors; and to our patients for inspiring us and reminding us of the urgency of our research."

Malouf's Dedication:
"I would like to dedicate this book to my mother Chams for her eternal love and infinite support, to the patients and their families, and to my co-editor Nizar Tannir for guiding my first steps in kidney cancer research as well as for his sincere friendship all along the road."

Preface

In recent years, researchers have made significant progress in the treatment of metastatic clear-cell renal cell carcinoma (ccRCC). Patients with ccRCC now benefit from a range of therapeutic options. However, advances in the treatment of rare, non-clear cell RCC variants have lagged behind those of their more common counterparts. Additionally, it is important to recognize that while these malignancies occur less frequently than ccRCC in the general population, they are the predominant variants in specific, often vulnerable, populations. For example, translocation RCC is the most common kidney cancer among children and young adults, and renal medullary carcinoma (RMC) specifically afflicts individuals with sickle hemoglobinopathies such as sickle cell trait. These patients will benefit from ongoing research efforts to elucidate the biology of these rare kidney tumors and develop therapeutic strategies aimed at improving the outcomes of these patients.

Comprehensive biological profiling initiatives such as The Cancer Genome Atlas (TCGA) have led to an unprecedented understanding of the molecular underpinnings of papillary and chromophobe RCC, the two most common non-clear cell variants. Similar efforts are underway for many of the less common non-clear cell RCCs. Currently available targeted therapies against ccRCC were informed by biological insights gained from the study of hereditary von Hippel-Lindau disease, and in a similar manner, the study of hereditary syndromes associated with non-clear cell RCCs is enhancing our understanding of rare kidney tumors. These efforts can guide the development of targeted therapies and immunotherapy approaches tailored to each non-clear cell variant.

As more non-clear cell tumors are being recognized and incorporated into classification systems, our published clinical experience with these entities is growing. This includes case reports, retrospective analyses, and even a steady trickle of prospective clinical trials. Nevertheless, most published therapeutic clinical trials dedicated to non-clear cell RCC do not distinguish among different histological subtypes. However, as we learn more about the features shared among non-clear cell variants, and those unique to each one, current and upcoming clinical trials are becoming more specific. For example, there are now trials focused on targeting the MET pathway in papillary RCC and proteotoxic stress in RMC.

In this rapidly changing landscape, it can be daunting for busy clinicians to keep abreast of new developments in the management of malignancies that are not part of their everyday repertoires. This book is intended to provide practicing clinicians and trainees with a concise overview of the biology, clinical presentation, diagnostic approaches, and treatment of rare kidney tumors. We hope that the information provided herein will benefit patients suffering from these diseases.

Strasbourg, France   Gabriel G. Malouf
Houston, TX   Nizar M. Tannir

Contents

Hereditary Renal Cell Carcinomas

Eric Jonasch and Patrick G. Pilie

Cancer initiation and progression is the result of an accumulation of mutations. Mutations occurring in cancer tissue are termed *somatic*, whereas mutations in germline DNA may be passed onto subsequent generations and are often termed *hereditary*. Deleterious germline mutations in key tumor suppressor genes can lead to hereditary cancer syndromes whereby family members carrying the mutation have an increased susceptibility to developing certain tumor phenotypes. Common features of hereditary cancer syndromes include early age of onset, multiple affected generations, rare tumor types, and/or multiple primary malignancies.

Renal cell carcinoma (RCC) is a diverse entity with variable histologic subtypes, and hereditary RCC, due to an inherited germline mutation, accounts for approximately 5 to 8% of all RCC cases, with variable penetrance depending on the gene mutated [1]. The majority of mutations in genes implicated in hereditary RCC are also seen in the significant majority of sporadic RCCs, such as *von Hippel-Lindau* (VHL) in clear cell RCC (ccRCC) and *MET* proto-oncogene in type 1 papillary RCC [2, 3]. Although distinct histologic subtypes of RCC exist, a shared feature across hereditary and sporadic RCC cases is dysregulation of the hypoxia-inducible factor (HIF) axis and aberrant tumor metabolism. In general, the median age of onset of hereditary RCC is 27 years younger than that observed for RCC in a general population, 37 years old versus 64 years old [1, 4]. If there is a concern for a hereditary RCC, the affected patient should be referred to a genetic counselor and tested for specific mutations based on the patient's personal medical and cancer history, family history, and RCC histology [4]. RCC that occurs in individuals 46 years old or younger may prompt referral to a genetic counselor and consideration for germline mutation testing regardless of family history or syndrome criteria [1].

E. Jonasch (✉) · P. G. Pilie
Department of Genitourinary Medical Oncology, The University of Texas MD Anderson
Cancer Center, Houston, TX, USA
e-mail: EJonasch@mdanderson.org

© Springer Nature Switzerland AG 2019   1
G. G. Malouf, N. M. Tannir (eds.), *Rare Kidney Tumors*,
https://doi.org/10.1007/978-3-319-96989-3_1

In this chapter, we will detail the various hereditary RCC syndromes and discuss genetic testing, cancer screening, and treatment in these unique populations.

1.1   von Hippel-Lindau Disease

Germline mutations in the von Hippel-Lindau (*VHL*) gene, a tumor suppressor found on chromosome 3p25, are inherited in an autosomal dominant fashion giving way to the potential development of a spectrum of tumor types including clear cell renal cell carcinoma (ccRCC), hemangioblastomas (HBs), pheochromocytomas, retinal hemangioblastomas, and pancreatic neuroendocrine tumors (pNETs) [5, 6]. Germline VHL mutations may be inherited from a parent or in rare cases due to de novo mutations occurring early on in embryogenesis. VHL disease occurs in approximately 1 in 35,000 births, and the morbidity and mortality associated with VHL disease center around the progression of ccRCC as well as the neurologic complications of hemangioblastomas [7]. The most common mutations seen in both sporadic and hereditary ccRCC are mutations in *VHL*. In general, individuals with ccRCC and a known family history of VHL or a VHL clinical phenotype, including bilateral or multifocal tumor presentation or a family history of renal tumors, should warrant *VHL* gene mutation testing [4]. Previous studies have shown that the specific type of genotypic alteration in the *VHL* gene may give way to the variance of phenotypic outcomes across families and individuals with VHL disease [8, 9]. Recommended surveillance for persons with known *VHL* germline mutations includes annual abdominal imaging and a central nervous system MRI every other year, annual audiometry and ophthalmologic exam, and annual laboratory work to include plasma metanephrines and chromogranin.

VHL disease-related lesions are in general highly vascular owing to the loss of the underlying anti-angiogenic function of the *VHL* gene product [7, 10]. The main function of the *VHL* gene product, pVHL, is to act as an oxygen sensor as part of the ubiquitin ligase E3 complex in normoxic conditions. pVHL exists as two domains, α and β, and forms a ternary complex with the transcription elongation factors C and B, which aid in stabilizing pVHL. This pVHL complex recognizes hydroxylated HIF-1α and HIF-2α and leads to the HIFs' proteosomal degradation. Without pVHL activity, as is the case in hypoxic conditions and VHL syndrome, HIF-1α and HIF-2α are allowed to transactivate their downstream pro-angiogenic elements, such as VEGF, PDGF, FGF, and GLUT1 and 3 in an unchecked manner. In the setting of pVHL loss, inhibition of HIF-2α is sufficient to suppress tumor formation [11]. pVHL also has non-HIF-related functions including key roles in extracellular matrix assembly, cilia maintenance, apoptosis regulation, genomic stability, and DNA damage repair [10, 12–14].

Given the variety of tumor types within a single individual with VHL disease, treatment necessitates a personalized, multidisciplinary approach; and given that the most frequent alterations in sporadic ccRCC involve the loss of the 3p chromosomal arm including the *VHL* gene, treatment discoveries for this rare, heritable disease have implications for a much wider patient population [2]. The primary treatment of VHL-associated lesions is surgical. HBs are the most frequently seen lesion in VHL disease, occurring in over 70% of patients. The next most frequent lesions include renal cysts and ccRCC tumors which occur in up to 60% of patients with VHL disease and often present as bilateral or multifocal disease [7]. Patients with known *VHL* mutations should undergo regular surveillance imaging including annual abdominal imaging for the presence of ccRCC. If discovered on surveillance imaging, RCC lesions are then monitored until the largest solid kidney tumor measures 3 cm or greater, which should prompt surgical intervention to prevent metastasis [15]. Once surgery is indicated, the goal is to preserve kidney function via a nephron-sparing approach and minimize surgical interventions and their associated morbidity as much as possible. Prior studies have shown that only 3% or fewer of patients with hereditary renal cell cancers undergoing repeat or salvage renal surgery progress to needing hemodialysis [16]. In general, the surgeon's desire to preserve kidney function in VHL-associated ccRCC is not different than in sporadic cases; but nephron-sparing is particularly important in hereditary kidney cancer populations given its typical earlier age of onset and bilateral or multifocal presentations necessitating multiple surgeries.

Patients with VHL disease with ccRCC will inevitably have progressively growing lesions or multiple synchronous tumors making surgical approaches difficult or contraindicated. Systemic treatment options for VHL-related ccRCC do not differ from those treatment options for sporadic cases at this time. Given that pVHL inactivation leads to inappropriate angiogenesis, tyrosine kinase inhibitors (TKIs) such as sunitinib, pazopanib, and cabozantinib directed against VEGF and other pro-angiogenic pathways are approved for metastatic ccRCC in sporadic and hereditary cases. A pilot study of sunitinib in 15 patients with germline *VHL* mutations with measurable VHL disease-associated lesions showed the drug had acceptable toxicity and 33% (6/18) of RCC lesions showed a partial response [17]. RCC in the endothelium displayed higher levels of pVEGFR-2 expression when compared to HBs, and interestingly, 0/21 HB lesions showed response to treatment with sunitinib. However, immunohistochemical expression levels of phosphorylated FGFR substrate 2 were higher in HBs, highlighting the heterogeneous nature of VHL-related lesions. A pilot trial of dovitinib, an inhibitor of VEGF and FGF signaling, was undertaken in patients with VHL syndrome and measurable HB lesion; however, the study drug yielded only stable disease as best response and was associated with significant toxicities [18]. A prior case study has shown that VHL-associated HBs can respond to pazopanib with reduction in size and symptoms, leading to a phase II trial of pazopanib in VHL syndrome patients with measureable lesions, which has shown early promising results with significant and sustained disease control in a number of VHL patients enrolled on the study [19]. Currently, if there is evidence of metastatic ccRCC in VHL patients, treatment approaches are the same as those in sporadic disease, which are evolving and may include multiple TKIs and/or immune checkpoint inhibition. A recent study that sequenced multiple ccRCCs from patients with *VHL* germline mutations has shown that even multiple tumors within a single individual display somatic heterogeneity and clonal independence [20]. There is no medical therapy that has been identified that works in all patients with VHL disease or even on all lesions within the same patient. Lastly, there are currently no preventative agents targeted or otherwise in use for prevention of VHL-related lesions.

1.2 Tuberous Sclerosis Complex Syndrome

Germline mutations in *TSC1/2* genes, located on chromosomes 9q34 and 16p13, respectively, can lead to a syndrome known as tuberous sclerosis complex (TSC) syndrome, which is inherited in an autosomal dominant fashion or may occur sporadically. The prevalence of TSC syndrome worldwide is approximately one million affected individuals. Clinically TSC syndrome is characterized by hamartomas and angiomyolipomas, which may spontaneously hemorrhage, as well as pulmonary lymphangioleiomyomatosis, subependymal giant cell astrocytomas, and RCC [7]. RCC in TSC syndrome is typically ccRCC in *TSC1* mutation carriers, but chromophobe histology is also seen in *TSC2* carriers, and *TSC2* is also mutated in sporadic chromophobe RCC [21]. In addition, as is seen in VHL disease, patients with TSC syndrome may develop kidney cysts associated with ciliary dysfunction. Typically, patients with TSC syndrome will develop multiple renal cysts and angiomyolipomas, which can invade adjacent renal parenchyma and lead to chronic kidney disease and ultimately death in this population [22].

Germline testing for *TSC1/2* mutations should be prompted based on clinical history, physical exam, and family history. Kidney cancer is not typically seen as a singular presentation of TSC syndrome. Active surveillance in patients with TSC syndrome should include brain and abdominal imaging every 1–3 years, chest imaging every 2–3 years, and an annual dermatologic exam. In addition, patients should undergo dental evaluation regularly, and an echocardiogram should be performed every 1–3 years.

TSC1 (hamartin) and *TSC2* (tuberin) form a heterodimer that works as a tumor suppressor to regulate mTOR complex 1 signaling cascade. *TSC1/2* mutations lead to mTORC1 dysregulation and overexpression, which aids cancer cells in proliferation, cytoskeletal rearrangements, nutrient excess, and protein synthesis [23]. Clinical trials using mTOR inhibitors in TSC syndrome patients showed efficacy, with a 42% response rate seen with everolimus, leading to its FDA approval for angiomyolipoma associated with TSC syndrome [23]. The majority of patients in this study had bilateral angiomyolipomas and 40% had invasive procedures; thus, everolimus should be considered in patients who are not surgical candidates and/or those with multifocal disease.

1.3 Phosphatase and Tensin Homolog Hamartoma Syndrome

Phosphatase and tensin homolog (*PTEN*) is a well-known tumor suppressor gene located on chromosome 10q23 and is responsible for AKT suppression and is integral in DNA damage repair. *PTEN* somatic mutations are seen in approximately 5%

of sporadic RCCs with posttranslational loss of PTEN protein expression seen frequently in RCC [2]. Deleterious germline mutations in *PTEN* give way to the PTEN hamartoma syndrome, a hereditary cancer disorder which is characterized by mucocutaneous lesions and cutaneous hamartomas as well as breast cancer, endometrial cancer, melanoma, and follicular thyroid cancer. Individuals with *PTEN* germline mutations have an approximately 34% lifetime risk of RCC, and RCC onset is typically at a younger than average age (~40 years old) [24]. Multiple case reports have shown the mTOR inhibitor sirolimus may be effective in individuals with PTEN hamartoma syndrome, and a clinical trial (NCT00971789) was completed but not yet reported [25, 26].

1.4 Succinate Dehydrogenase-Associated Renal Cell Carcinoma

Rare germline mutations in the tricarboxylic acid cycle (Krebs) gene, succinate dehydrogenase (*SDH*), can give way to a multiple primary tumor phenotype that may include ccRCC. *SDH* is a family of genes including *SDHA, SDHB, SDHC,* and *SDHD*. Germline mutations in *SDHB* were first described in families with RCC and/or hereditary paragangliomas or gastrointestinal stromal tumors, though RCC may be the only clinical manifestation in individuals with germline *SDHB, SDHC,* and *SDHD* genes. In small, family-based retrospective studies, the mean and median age of SDHB-associated RCC was 33 and 30 years, respectively [27]. *SDHB/C/D* germline mutation testing may be considered in patients with early-onset RCC or for those with a family history of RCC and/or paragangliomas and pheochromocytomas. There are no guidelines for surveillance, but yearly abdominal imaging for RCC should be considered.

SDH is a key enzyme in the Krebs cycle, and mutations in *SDH* subunits cause accumulation of succinate as well as inhibition of proly hydroxylation of HIF-1α and HIF-2α. Cells with mutated Krebs cycle enzymes exhibit increased glucose uptake, aerobic glycolysis, and fatty acid synthesis, which are also known as the Warburg effect. Thus, targeting these metabolic shifts may be particularly suited for *SDH* mutant-related RCC.

1.5 Hereditary Papillary Renal Cell Carcinoma and Hereditary Leiomyomatosis and RCC

Papillary renal cell carcinoma is the second most common histologic subtype, accounting for 15–20% of RCC. Two major subtypes of papillary RCC exist, including type 1 and type 2, and these subtypes have distinct genetic alterations and associated hereditary syndromes.

Hereditary papillary RCC (HPRC) or type 1 papillary RCC is an autosomal dominant cancer syndrome due to mutations in the proto-oncogene *MET* on chromosome 7q31, with somatic *MET* mutations found in 13–15% of sporadic papillary RCC [3, 28]. Persons with HPRC syndrome typically display multiple tumors in bilateral kidneys, and extrarenal manifestations are not reported. However, metastatic potential of these tumors is low. Active surveillance with annual CT/MRI abdominal imaging is recommended, and nephron-sparing surgery is considered when a tumor reaches 3 cm or greater to mitigate risk of metastatic disease while preserving renal function.

The *MET* gene product is a cell surface receptor protein for hepatocyte growth factor (HGF) which promotes tumor cell migration, invasion, proliferation, and angiogenesis. A phase II study of the MET/VEGFR2 inhibitor, foretinib, was performed in 74 patients with papillary RCC, including 11 patients with pathogenic germline *MET* mutations. In this trial, objective response rate (ORR) was 13.5% with ten responders achieving a partial response (PR) only. Analysis based on germline *MET* mutational status revealed that 50% of germline carriers achieved a PR, while only 9% of those patients without a germline mutation achieved a PR [29].

Type 2 papillary RCC is a heterogeneous disease with multiple subtypes. Germline mutations in the fumarate hydratase (*FH*) gene on chromosome 1q42 give way to aggressive type 2 tumors seen in the context of hereditary leiomyomatosis and RCC (HLRCC) syndrome. The clinical phenotype of HLRCC syndrome typically includes cutaneous and/or uterine leiomyomas and type 2 papillary RCC. The median age of onset for papillary RCC in this population is 37 years, and surveillance should include dermatologic evaluation every 1–2 years, annual abdominal MRI, and annual gynecologic exam and ultrasound. Given the aggressive nature of the type 2 papillary RCC in HLRCC syndrome, immediate surgery for an identified renal tumor is warranted rather than the typical 3 cm size threshold used in other hereditary renal syndromes. Fumarate hydratase is a Krebs cycle enzyme that converts fumarate to malate. *FH* biallelic inactivation in HLRCC syndrome results in complete loss or reduction of the FH enzymatic activity which then leads to intracellular fumarate accumulation and a metabolic shift to aerobic glycolysis, termed the Warburg effect [30, 31]. Combination therapy targeting VEGFR and EGFR using bevacizumab in conjunction with erlotinib has been shown to have activity against familial type 2 papillary RCC in HLRCC syndrome, and a prospective phase II trial is underway (NCT01130519) [32]. In addition, a clinical trial using vandetanib, a multikinase inhibitor including targets VEGFR and EGFR, in combination with metformin is underway (NCT02495103) for patients with advanced HLRCC and sporadic papillary RCC.

1.6   Birt-Hogg-Dubé

Birt-Hogg-Dubé (BHD) is an autosomal dominant syndrome characterized by fibrofolliculomas, pulmonary cysts, and/or renal lesions, typically oncocytomas or chromophobe RCC. The risk of developing RCC in patients with BHD is estimated to be 16% by age 70, and BHD patients have a 50-fold increased risk of developing a pneumothorax across age groups. BHD is the result of germline loss-of-function mutations in folliculin (*FLCN*) gene found on chromosome 17p11, with hotspot mutation areas in exons 11–13 [33, 34]. The FLCN gene product is downstream of mTORC1 signaling and localizes to cilia. Loss of FLCN function leads to mTORC1 activation and dysregulated ciliogenesis. Single allele loss leading to haploinsufficiency is enough to lead to skin manifestations of BHD, while biallelic loss is required for the development of RCC lesions [34].

Surveillance of patients with known *FLCN* germline mutations should include yearly abdominal imaging. In addition, given the risk of pulmonary cysts and pneumothorax, patients with BHD should have consultation with a pulmonologist stressing risk reduction strategies and smoking cessation if applicable [35].

Similar to most other hereditary RCC syndromes, active surveillance of renal lesions should be performed until a lesion reaches a size of 3 cm, at which time nephron-sparing resection is recommended. Preclinical data has suggested mTOR inhibition is effective at prolonging survival in FLCN-deficient mice; however, a clinical trial of topical rapamycin for BHD-associated fibrofolliculomas did not reduce size or burden of cutaneous lesions. Due to the rarity of this syndrome and its associated tumors, tailored treatment strategies are lacking, and thus, multi-institutional, global partnered trials are crucial.

1.7   BRCA1-Associated Protein-1 Predisposition to Familial ccRCC

Approximately 5–15% of sporadic ccRCCs show loss-of-function mutations in the BRCA1-associated protein-1 (*BAP1*), a gene which resides on chromosome 3p21.1 [36]. BAP1 protein functions as a nuclear deubiquitinase that interacts with polycomb group proteins at open chromatin and promotes double-strand break repair. Germline mutations in *BAP1* have been seen in association with familial ccRCC in addition to other cancers including uveal melanoma, malignant mesothelioma, and cutaneous melanoma; however, the prevalence of BAP1 syndrome and the associated risk of RCC are not well understood due to its rarity [37]. Like other familial cancer syndromes, cancers associated with *BAP1* germline mutations seem to have early age of onset and more aggressive phenotypes [38]. Early-onset RCC screening may be pursued based on the age of initial presentation of ccRCC.

Conclusions

Hereditary cancers account for approximately 10% of all cancers including RCC. Populations with hereditary cancer syndromes present unique challenges to oncology healthcare teams including risk assessment, counseling, surveillance, and therapeutic management. A thorough family and personal medical history in combination with a patient's RCC histology and phenotypic presentation will help guide genetic testing and interpretation. If a pathogenic germline mutation is discovered, then tailored surveillance and intervention strategies should be followed. A proband's family members should then be counseled on their own risk of carrying the pathogenic variant and can decide on genetic testing with the help of a certified genetic counselor. Unaffected carriers should undergo specified surveillance as early detection is currently the only clinically available prevention strategy for hereditary RCC syndromes. As noted, there is considerable overlap between gene mutations in hereditary and sporadic RCC, and research into these rare hereditary cancer syndromes has greatly informed the understanding of RCC tumorigenesis as a whole [2, 3, 21]. Despite the varied, complex pathways involved in hereditary RCC syndromes, they share a common dysregulation of the HIF-VEGF axis coupled with aberrant tumor metabolism which offers targetable pathways for precision medicine approaches in RCC syndromes. There is ongoing research into alternative treatment strategies to improve the targeting of VEGF or mTOR pathways as well as identify new druggable targets for the treatment of the varied RCC histologies. As with all hereditary cancer syndromes, targeted prevention strategies coupled with improved biomarkers for early detection and treatment monitoring are needed to make a significant impact on quality of life and long-term survival in RCC patients with pathogenic germline mutations and their family members who are unaffected carriers. With paired germline and somatic next-generation sequencing becoming ubiquitous across major cancer centers, it is likely that novel mutations may be discovered that are associated with hereditary RCC syndromes [39]. It is important particularly in these rare cancer syndromes that the medical community work together to qualify and quantify the genotype-phenotype correlations associated with these pathogenic germline mutations so that we can improve upon risk stratification, prevention, surveillance, and treatment for our patients and their families.

References

1. Shuch B, Vourganti S, Ricketts CJ, et al. Defining early-onset kidney cancer: implications for germline and somatic mutation testing and clinical management. J Clin Oncol. 2014;32:431–7.
2. Cancer Genome Atlas Research Network. Comprehensive molecular characterization of clear cell renal cell carcinoma. Nature. 2013;499:43–9.
3. Cancer Genome Atlas Research Network, Linehan WM, Spellman PT, et al. Comprehensive Molecular Characterization of Papillary Renal-Cell Carcinoma. N Engl J Med. 2016;374:135–45.
4. Linehan WM. Evaluation and screening for hereditary renal cell cancers. Can Urol Assoc J. 2013;7:324–5.
5. Latif F, Tory K, Gnarra J, et al. Identification of the von Hippel-Lindau disease tumor suppressor gene. Science. 1993;260:1317–20.
6. Butman JA, Linehan WM, Lonser RR. Neurologic manifestations of von Hippel-Lindau disease. JAMA. 2008;300:1334–42.
7. Ho TH, Jonasch E. Genetic kidney cancer syndromes. J Natl Compr Cancer Netw. 2014;12:1347–55.
8. McNeill A, Rattenberry E, Barber R, et al. Genotype-phenotype correlations in VHL exon deletions. Am J Med Genet A. 2009;149A:2147–51.
9. Lonser RR, Butman JA, Huntoon K, et al. Prospective natural history study of central nervous system hemangioblastomas in von Hippel-Lindau disease. J Neurosurg. 2014;120:1055–62.
10. Gossage L, Eisen T, Maher ER. VHL, the story of a tumour suppressor gene. Nat Rev Cancer. 2015;15:55–64.

11. Kondo K, Kim WY, Lechpammer M, et al. Inhibition of HIF2alpha is sufficient to suppress pVHL-defective tumor growth. PLoS Biol. 2003;1:E83.
12. Thoma CR, Frew IJ, Hoerner CR, et al. pVHL and GSK3beta are components of a primary cilium-maintenance signalling network. Nat Cell Biol. 2007;9:588–95.
13. Ding X-F, Zhou J, Hu Q-Y, et al. The tumor suppressor pVHL down-regulates never-in-mitosis A-related kinase 8 via hypoxia-inducible factors to maintain cilia in human renal cancer cells. J Biol Chem. 2015;290:1389–94.
14. Metcalf JL, Bradshaw PS, Komosa M, et al. K63-ubiquitylation of VHL by SOCS1 mediates DNA double-strand break repair. Oncogene. 2014;33:1055–65.
15. Duffey BG, Choyke PL, Glenn G, et al. The relationship between renal tumor size and metastases in patients with von Hippel-Lindau disease. J Urol. 2004;172:63–5.
16. Metwalli AR, Linehan WM. Nephron-sparing surgery for multifocal and hereditary renal tumors. Curr Opin Urol. 2014;24:466–73.
17. Jonasch E, McCutcheon IE, Waguespack SG, et al. Pilot trial of sunitinib therapy in patients with von Hippel-Lindau disease. Ann Oncol. 2011;22:2661–6.
18. Pilie PG, Matin SF, Woodson AH, et al. Pilot study of dovitinib in patients with VHL disease. J Clin Oncol. 2016;34:587.
19. Jonasch E, Gombos DS, Waguespack SG, et al. Phase II study of pazopanib in patients with von Hippel-Lindau disease. J Clin Oncol. 2017;35:4516.
20. Fei SS, Mitchell AD, Heskett MB, et al. Patient-specific factors influence somatic variation patterns in von Hippel-Lindau disease renal tumours. Nat Commun. 2016;7:11588.
21. The .somatic genomic landscape of chromophobe renal cell carcinoma. – PubMed – NCBI. 2018. https://www.ncbi.nlm.nih.gov/pubmed/25155756?dopt=Abstract. Cited 2018 Mar 22.
22. Shepherd CW, Gomez MR, Lie JT, et al. Causes of death in patients with tuberous sclerosis. Mayo Clin Proc. 1991;66:792–6.
23. Bissler JJ, Kingswood JC, Radzikowska E, et al. Everolimus for angiomyolipoma associated with tuberous sclerosis complex or sporadic lymphangioleiomyomatosis (EXIST-2): a multicentre, randomised, double-blind, placebo-controlled trial. Lancet. 2013;381:817–24.
24. Tan M-H, Mester JL, Ngeow J, et al. Lifetime cancer risks in individuals with germline PTEN mutations. Clin Cancer Res. 2012;18:400–7.
25. Marsh DJ, Trahair TN, Martin JL, et al. Rapamycin treatment for a child with germline PTEN mutation. Nat Clin Pract Oncol. 2008;5:357–61.
26. Schmid GL, Kässner F, Uhlig HH, et al. Sirolimus treatment of severe PTEN hamartoma tumor syndrome: case report and in vitro studies. Pediatr Res. 2014;75:527–34.
27. Ricketts CJ, Shuch B, Vocke CD, et al. Succinate Dehydrogenase Kidney Cancer (SDH-RCC): An Aggressive Example of the Warburg Effect in Cancer. J Urol. 2012;188:2063–71. http://www.ncbi.nlm.nih.gov/pmc/articles/PMC3856891/. Cited 2016 Nov 12
28. Schmidt L, Duh FM, Chen F, et al. Germline and somatic mutations in the tyrosine kinase domain of the MET proto-oncogene in papillary renal carcinomas. Nat Genet. 1997;16:68–73.
29. Choueiri TK, Vaishampayan U, Rosenberg JE, et al. Phase II and biomarker study of the dual MET/VEGFR2 inhibitor foretinib in patients with papillary renal cell carcinoma. J Clin Oncol. 2013;31:181–6.
30. Vocke CD, Ricketts CJ, Merino MJ, et al. Comprehensive genomic and phenotypic characterization of germline FH deletion in hereditary leiomyomatosis and renal cell carcinoma. Genes Chromosomes Cancer. 2017;56:484–92.
31. Menko FH, Maher ER, Schmidt LS, et al. Hereditary leiomyomatosis and renal cell cancer (HLRCC): renal cancer risk, surveillance and treatment. Familial Cancer. 2014;13:637–44.
32. Modi PK, Singer EA. Improving our understanding of papillary renal cell carcinoma with integrative genomic analysis. Ann Transl Med. 2016;4:143. http://www.ncbi.nlm.nih.gov/pmc/articles/PMC4842405/. Cited 2016 Nov 11
33. Luijten MNH, Basten SG, Claessens T, et al. Birt-Hogg-Dube syndrome is a novel ciliopathy. Hum Mol Genet. 2013;22:4383–97.

34. Bratslavsky G, Woodford MR, Daneshvar M, et al. Sixth BHD Symposium and First International Upstate Kidney Cancer Symposium: latest scientific and clinical discoveries. Oncotarget. 2016;7:15292–8.
35. Johannesma PC, van de Beek I, van der Wel JWT, et al. Risk of spontaneous pneumothorax due to air travel and diving in patients with Birt-Hogg-Dubé syndrome. Springerplus. 2016;5:1506.
36. Yu H, Pak H, Hammond-Martel I, et al. Tumor suppressor and deubiquitinase BAP1 promotes DNA double-strand break repair. Proc Natl Acad Sci U S A. 2014;111:285–90.
37. Popova T, Hebert L, Jacquemin V, et al. Germline BAP1 mutations predispose to renal cell carcinomas. Am J Hum Genet. 2013;92:974–80.
38. Rai K, Pilarski R, Cebulla CM, et al. Comprehensive review of BAP1 tumor predisposition syndrome with report of two new cases. Clin Genet. 2016;89:285–94.
39. Mandelker D, Zhang L, Kemel Y, et al. Mutation Detection in Patients With Advanced Cancer by Universal Sequencing of Cancer-Related Genes in Tumor and Normal DNA vs Guideline-Based Germline Testing. JAMA. 2017;318:825–35.

Wilms Tumor-Nephroblastoma

Marie V. Nelson, Arnauld Verschuur, and Jeffrey S. Dome

2.1 Introduction

Nephroblastoma, or Wilms tumor (WT), is the second most common extracranial solid tumor and the most common malignant renal tumor in children, accounting for 5% of all malignancies and 80% of all diagnosed renal cancers in children and teenagers. The overall survival has increased to over 90% due to international collaboration in cooperative group studies and employment of a multimodal treatment approach including surgery, radiation, and chemotherapy [1, 2]. The earliest of these studies, led by the National Wilms Tumor Study Group (NWTSG), which was superseded by the Children's Oncology Group (COG) in 2002, and the International Society of Paediatric Oncology (SIOP), stratified patients based on tumor stage alone. However, over time, the discovery of additional clinical, histological, and biological prognostic factors has led to more precise treatments that augment therapy for patients at high risk of relapse while reducing therapy for patients at low risk of relapse.

The progress in outcome made over the last four decades has made WT one of the successes of Paediatric oncology and of modern medicine. Despite the success, more advancement is required, as certain patient subgroups continue to have high risk for tumor recurrence and death. As the molecular mechanisms and biology underlying WT are studied and better understood, there is hope that there will not only be more survivors in the future but survivors living healthier lives.

M. V. Nelson · J. S. Dome (✉)
Center for Cancer and Blood Disorders, Children's National Health System,
Washington, DC, USA
e-mail: jdome@childrensnational.org

A. Verschuur
Centre de Cancérologie Pédiatrique, Hôpital d'Enfants de la Timone,
Marseille, France

© Springer Nature Switzerland AG 2019
G. Malouf, N. M. Tannir (eds.), *Rare Kidney Tumors*,
https://doi.org/10.1007/978-3-319-96989-3_2

WT is a malignancy with a rich historical background that not only unites the disciplines of development and genetics but also surgery, radiation therapy, and oncology in its treatment. The following pages review the epidemiology and pathogenesis, presentation, important prognostic factors, treatment, outcome, and future directions of research and therapy of WT.

2.2   Pathogenesis and Epidemiology

WT is a malignant embryonal tumor of young children, with most cases diagnosed in children under the age of 5 years. In the United States and Canada, the estimated incidence is 9.0 per million, affecting 1 in 10,000 children [3, 4]. Similar rates have been reported in Europe, Australia, and New Zealand, with lower rates in Asia and Central and South America, while in areas of Africa, such as Harare, Zimbabwe, the incidence is as high as 16.5 per million [3]. The diagnosis of WT is extraordinarily rare in adults, with incidence of only 0.2 cases per million [5].

WT was first described in 1899, when Max Wilms established the classical description of a "mixed tumor," comprised of epithelial, blastemal, and stromal cells [6, 7]. He hypothesized that WT cells arose from a common, undifferentiated renal cell, which has since been supported, holding that WT evolution is rooted in normal kidney development. During development, the fetal kidney arises from the ureteric bud which forms the collecting ducts and the metanephric mesenchyme or blastema which forms the stroma and the other tubular structures, including the glomeruli, proximal and distal tubules, and loop of Henle [8]. While the blastemal component usually disappears by 36-week gestation, 1% of infants will retain these collections of embryonic cells, referred to as "nephrogenic rests." Nephrogenic rests are potentially precursor lesions of WT and can be found in 40% of patients, and over 90% of patients with bilateral disease, suggesting a germline mutation may predispose to the persistence of such rests. Most cases of WT are unilateral, with 5–10% of cases affecting both kidneys. Bilateral WT is more common in patients with underlying genetic syndromes.

More than 15 different syndromes are associated with WT, including WAGR (Wilms tumor, aniridia, genitourinary abnormalities, and mental retardation), Denys-Drash (Wilms tumor, diffuse mesangial sclerosis leading to early-onset renal failure, and intersex disorders that can range from ambiguous to normal-appearing female genitalia in both XY and XX individuals), and Beckwith-Wiedemann (embryonal tumors, macrosomia, macroglossia, hemihypertrophy, visceromegaly, omphalocele, neonatal hypoglycemia, and ear creases/pits) [9]. Less than 5% of WT cases are associated with an underlying syndrome, and therefore, the etiology of most cases is unknown. However, a strong genetic contribution is suggested given that geographical variation is closely linked to ancestry and that 2% of WT cases are familial [10].

Beckwith–Wiedemann Syndrome (BWS), the most common overgrowth syndrome, and isolated hemihypertrophy are associated with genetic or epigenetic abnormalities in the 11p15 region [11–13]. A number of imprinted genes have been identified in this region, including *IGF2*, *H19*, and *CDKN1C*, though *IGF2* has been most clearly implicated in WT development. In normal cells, *IGF2* is expressed only from the paternal allele. In WT, two primary mechanisms lead to *IGF2* overexpression with roughly equal frequency: uniparental isodisomy, which is the duplication of the paternally derived chromosome, and loss of imprinting (LOI), which results from hypermethylation and expression from the normally silent maternal allele. The risk of WT and other embryonal tumors in BWS is about 5–10%, though molecular phenotypes of BWS involving *IGF2* overexpression carry a risk of nearly 40% [14]. Approximately 70% of WT overexpress *IGF2*, even in the absence of BWS or hemihypertophy [13].

Mutations in the *WT1* gene, located at 11p13, are associated with a number of WT predisposition syndromes, including WAGR, in which a large deletion of the *WT1* gene is present. Mutations in *WT1* can also be seen in Frasier syndrome and Denys-Drash syndrome (DDS). *WT1*, a tumor suppressor gene, was the first described gene in the development of WT. *WT1* codes for a zinc finger transcription factor crucial for the mesenchymal-to-epithelial transition in kidney development and is highly expressed in the developing kidney, gonads, and spleen [12, 15]. The type of mutation (protein truncation, deletion, or missense mutation) affects the clinical phenotype, including genitourinary anomalies, renal failure, and cancer risk, and while mutations in *WT1* are well-described in syndromes discussed above, they are only present in 10–20% of sporadic WT. Incidence of WT differs among these syndromes, at 45 to 50% in patients with known *WT1* deletion and 75% in patients with DDS.

Mutations within the WNT signaling pathway have also been well-described in WT literature. Activating mutations of *CTNNB1*, the gene that encodes the β-catenin protein, a central effector of the WNT pathway, have been identified in about 15% of WTs [16, 17]. There is a strong correlation between *CTNNB1* mutations and *WT1* mutations, suggesting a cooperative effect between these two pathways. Alterations in another gene, *AMER1* (also known as *WTX*), encoding another component of the WNT signaling pathway, have been found in up to 33% of WT [18–20].

More recently, genes involved in microRNA (miRNA) biogenesis were discovered in approximately 15% of Wilms tumors. Genes encoding proteins that operate at various points in the miRNA processing pathway, including *DROSHA*, *DGCR8*, *DICER1*, *XPO5*, *TARBP2*, and *DISL32*, were found to be mutated in WT, some associated with high-risk blastemal tumors [21–24]. The miRNA gene mutations impair the generation of mature tumor suppressing miRNAs including let-7, which is involved in renal tumor development. Recently, mutations in the renal development genes *SIX1* and *SIX2* have been observed in approximately 5% of WT [21, 22]. Mutations in *MLLT1*, which encodes a component of the RNA super elongation complex, have been observed in approximately 10% of WT [25]. As more is discovered regarding the intricate genetic mystery underlying WT, the complex heterogeneity of this tumor is also realized, uncovering the need for additional research.

2.3 Diagnosis

2.3.1 History and Physical

The initial presentation of WT is usually asymptomatic; the parent may identify an abdominal mass on bathing or dressing the child, or the Paediatrician may palpate the mass upon examining the child during their routine well-child visit. The patient is usually asymptomatic; however, up to 35% of patients can present with either hematuria, hypertension, fever, or flank pain [26]. In rare cases, a patient may have the severe presentation of an acute abdomen in the setting of tumor rupture and bleeding into the surrounding tissue, which can be associated with extreme pain and anemia.

The differential diagnosis includes other renal malignancies such as renal cell carcinoma (which is typically seen in adolescents and adults), clear cell sarcoma of the kidney, rhabdoid tumor, and congenital mesoblastic nephroma, as well as benign renal masses such as renal cysts or dysplastic kidneys. Neuroblastoma, which can arise from the adrenal gland, is a more common malignant abdominal tumor found in the same age group and should be considered. Patients with neuroblastoma tend to be symptomatic and sometimes ill-appearing at diagnosis contrasted with WT patients who are mostly well-appearing and asymptomatic.

A thorough history should be taken, with attention to history of cancer predisposition, congenital anomalies, or urogenital defects, as well as the child's birth and developmental history. Physical exam should include blood pressure measurement due to risk of hypertension, and examination for physical malformations should be done to assess for WT-related syndromes. Findings on exam are a firm, non-tender mass which usually does not cross the midline of the patient [27].

2.3.2 Imaging and Laboratory Findings

In the setting of a clinical suspicion, ultrasound (US) with Doppler is an effective imaging modality to assess for an abdominal mass, determine its characteristics (cystic, solid, vascular), and evaluate site of origin and extent into the renal vein and inferior vena cava. If ultrasound reveals a renal mass, computed tomography (CT) scan or magnetic resonance imaging (MRI) is then used to evaluate the origin and extent of the tumor and the presence of contralateral renal tumors to assist in surgical planning. The COG performed a study comparing the two modalities and found that CT and MRI had similar diagnostic performance in detection of lymph node involvement and capsular spread. MRI was more likely to reveal contralateral disease, however only in a small number of patients. Therefore, either modality was deemed appropriate in diagnosis [26, 27].

Imaging is also important to survey the chest for pulmonary metastasis, the most common location for distant disease, present in up to 10–20% of cases. Previously, plain radiographs were used to evaluate for thoracic metastasis but now have been mostly replaced by CT scan [28]. CT scans are more sensitive in detecting small lung nodules, but this has created uncertainty regarding the optimal definition and treatment of pulmonary metastatic disease. Up to 25% of pulmonary nodules less than 1 cm that have been biopsied were benign, and there is considerable inter-reader variability among radiologists in detecting sub-centimeter nodules [29, 30]. However, studies have shown that patients who have small nodules visualized on CT scan have inferior event-free and/or overall survival compared to patients without nodules, especially when the treatment does not include doxorubicin [28, 31, 32]. This suggests that CT scans add prognostic value and that small nodules should not be disregarded. However, through cooperative group clinic trials, we have discovered that not all patients with pulmonary disease require chest radiation, as will be discussed in a later section.

Laboratory testing, while not diagnostic in WT, is important nonetheless. Patients with suspected renal masses should have a complete blood count and a complete metabolic panel to evaluate renal and liver function. Coagulation studies and blood type and screen are usually completed prior to surgical intervention. WT has been rarely associated with von Willebrand disease, a bleeding disorder related to primary hemostasis [33]. Urinary catecholamine studies are recommended on SIOP protocols to evaluate for neuroblastoma.

2.3.3   Histopathology

While age of patient, clinical and laboratory features, and imaging characteristics are undoubtedly helpful in making the diagnosis of WT, the gold standard remains histologic assessment of the tumor. Remarkable histologic diversity is present among these tumors, with the classic description of WT being of triphasic morphology, including blastemal, stromal, and epithelial elements. A variety of cell types can be identified within the tumor, including skeletal muscle, cartilage, and squamous epithelium, hypothesized to be due to pluripotent potential of the metanephric blastemal cell from which the tumor arises [34].

Nephrogenic rests are remnants of renal embryonal tissue that are considered precursor lesions to WT and are found in 30–40% of patients [34]. Two distinct entities of nephrogenic rests have been identified. Perilobar nephrogenic rests (PLNR) are found at the periphery of the renal lobe, more numerous in quantity, and associated with older age at diagnosis and hemihypertrophy. They are less likely to evolve into WT. Intralobar nephrogenic rests (ILNR) are associated with younger age at diagnosis and presence of aniridia, GU abnormalities, and bilateral disease [34].

2.4   Prognostic Factors

2.4.1   Tumor Stage

Tumor stage is one of the most important prognostic factors for WT [2]. Locoregional tumor extension and distant metastasis correlate with higher-stage disease, inferior prognosis, and higher risk of recurrence in comparison to disease limited to the kidney. The presence/absence of metastatic disease denoting stage IV disease is made based on initial imaging, but local (abdominal) tumor stage is also an important factor. The COG staging system is based on clinical and pathological features before chemotherapy is given. Most patients treated according to COG protocols undergo immediate nephrectomy, at which time a local stage is assigned. If a patient receives chemotherapy before nephrectomy, the tumor is automatically classified as stage III. By contrast, the staging system used by the SIOP is based on stage after 4 to 6 weeks of preoperative chemotherapy [2]. Despite these important differences, the two systems have common features that lead to a designation of stage III, including tumor at the surgical margin, tumor rupture, peritoneal implants, and positive lymph nodes [2, 35]. The current COG and SIOP staging systems are found in Table 2.1.

Table 2.1 Comparison of renal tumor staging systems: COG and SIOP approaches

Stage	COG	SIOP
I	• Tumor confined to the kidney • Renal capsule intact • Tumor completely resected • No involvement of renal sinus vessels • No biopsy performed • No tumor beyond surgical margins	• Tumor confined to the kidney or is surrounded by fibrous pseudocapsule and is completely resected • No involvement of renal sinus vessels • Necrotic tumor in the renal sinus or perirenal fat does not upstage to stage II as long as it does not reach the resection margins • Percutaneous cutting needle biopsy allowed
II	• Tumor extension beyond the kidney and/or penetration of renal capsule but completely resected • Local invasion of adjacent structures or extension into the vena cava is allowed as long as resected en bloc with no evidence of tumor at or beyond margins • No tumor rupture of spillage • No biopsy performed	• Tumor extension beyond the kidney or renal pseudocapsule but completely resected • Infiltration of renal sinus and/or blood and lymphatic vessels outside renal parenchyma but completely resected • Local invasion of adjacent structures or extension into the vena cava is allowed as long as resected en bloc with no evidence of tumor at or beyond margins
III	*Meeting one or multiple criteria below:* • Tumor extends to or beyond resection margins microscopically or there is macroscopic incomplete excision • Positive abdominal lymph nodes • Tumor rupture before or intraoperatively including spillage confined to the flank or diffuse peritoneal contamination by the tumor or where peritoneal implants are present • Fractional removal of tumor • Any biopsy performed prior to surgery OR tumor not resected prior to starting chemotherapy	*Meeting one or multiple criteria below:* • Tumor extends to or beyond resection margins microscopically or there is macroscopic incomplete excision • Positive abdominal lymph nodes • Tumor rupture before or intraoperatively including diffuse peritoneal contamination by the tumor or where peritoneal implants are present • Fractional removal of tumor • Open biopsy prior to preoperative chemotherapy or surgery
IV	• Presence of distant metastasis or lymph node involvement	• Presence of distant metastasis or lymph node involvement
V	• Bilateral renal involvement at diagnosis • Each tumor is substaged based on above system	• Bilateral renal involvement at diagnosis • Each tumor is substaged based on above system

COG Children's Oncology Group, *SIOP* International Society of Paediatric Oncology

2.4.2   Histology

Histology is undoubtedly the most powerful prognostic factor for WT [2]. Histologic risk categories for both COG and SIOP are found in Table 2.2. Anaplastic histology WT (AHWT) is a distinct subtype characterized by a morphologic presence of large polypoid nuclei at least three times that of adjacent cells, presence of mitotic figures, and hyperchromasia. The incidence of AHWT was found to be as high as 10.8% of all cases in National Wilms Tumor Study (NWTS)-5 and carries a poorer prognosis than favorable histology WT (FHWT) [36]. There is an undeniable link between *TP53* mutations and AHWT cells, as these mutations are mostly found in areas of anaplasia and very rarely in FHWT [37]. *TP53* mutations have been reported in anywhere between 50 and 86% of AHWT. Moreover, *TP53* mutation was recently found to be associated with a significantly increased risk of relapse and death in patients with stage III and stage IV AHWT versus those who had wild-type form of *TP53* (61% vs. 13%, respectively) [38]. These findings have spurred questions whether *TP53* mutation status should be used to determine treatment in AHWT.

2.4.3   Molecular Biology

The prospective goal of the NWTS-5 trial was to better understand the prognostic significance of loss of heterozygosity (LOH) for chromosomes 16q and 1p in FHWT, which in earlier studies appeared to be associated with worse outcome. LOH for either chromosome segment was found to correlate with increased risk of relapse and death in all stages; however, the most significant impact was in groups with LOH for both 16q and 1p. For stage I/II tumors, 4-year relapse-free survival (RFS) and overall survival (OS) were 91.2% and 98.4% for tumors without LOH, compared to 74.9% and 90.5% for tumors with combined LOH ($p = 0.001$ for RFS and 0.01 for OS). For stage III/IV tumors, 4-year RFS and OS were 83% and 91.9% for tumors without LOH,

Table 2.2   Histologic classification of Wilms tumor

International Society of Paediatric Oncology (SIOP)	Children's Oncology Group (COG)
Low-risk Wilms tumor	*Favorable histology Wilms tumor*
Completely necrotic	No evidence of anaplasia
Cystic, partially differentiated	
Intermediate-risk Wilms tumor	*Focal Anaplastic Wilms tumor*
Epithelial, stromal, mixed, or regressive types	Anaplasia confined to one or more circumscribed sites within the primary tumor, no extrarenal involvement
Focal anaplastic histology	No nuclear unrest outside of anaplastic areas
High-risk Wilms tumor	*Diffuse anaplastic Wilms tumor*
Blastemal type	Nonlocalized anaplasia
Diffuse anaplastic histology	Anaplasia in invasive sites, extrarenal involvement
	Localized anaplasia with severe nuclear unrest
	Anaplasia in random biopsy specimen or involving the edge of one or more sections

compared to 65.9% and 77.5% for tumors with combined LOH ($p = 0.01$ for RFS and 0.04 for OS) [39]. Due to these findings, patients with combined LOH at 16q and 1p receive augmented therapy according to the current COG risk stratification schema.

Gain of chromosome 1q is one of the most commonly found cytogenetic abnormalities found in WT, seen in as many as 30% of cases [40, 41]. Earlier studies have indicated that this anomaly was associated with lower event-free survival (EFS) and OS independent of tumor stage yet lacked substantial power. The NWTS-5 and SIOP studies have confirmed that 1q gain was associated with inferior EFS across all tumor stages and inferior OS in stage I and IV unilateral FHWT [40, 41]. There also was a correlation between LOH 16q/1p and gain of 1q because a translocation involving chromosomes 1p and 16q followed by duplication of chromosome 1 can give rise to LOH 1p and 16 as well as 1q gain [42]. Gain of 1q will likely be incorporated into the next treatment stratification in COG studies. In SIOP studies, 1q gain correlated with blastemal-type histology, which is already used for risk stratification.

2.4.4   Age

Previous trials have shown that increasing age of the patient is associated with increased risk of recurrence. This was formerly attributed to the fact that AHWT is rare in very young patients; however, older patients with FHWT do have a less favorable outcome than their younger counterparts [43]. Currently, according to the COG strategy, age is only incorporated into treatment stratification for patients less than 2 years of age with stage I FHWT and tumor weight less than or equal to 550 g. This small group of patients has a very good outcome with surgery alone with overall survival close to 100% [44–46]. Despite the fact that these very low-risk WT (VLRWT) patients in general have been found to do very well long term, recent studies have shown that VLRWT patients with LOH or LOI at 11p15 were at increased risk of relapse, suggesting that these biomarkers may be helpful in predicting those who may need adjuvant chemotherapy [46, 47].

2.5   Staging and Treatment

The overall survival rate in patients with WT has increased to over 90% due to clinical trials performed by a number of collaborative organizations, including the NWTSG, COG, SIOP, and other international groups [2]. The treatment of WT is multidisciplinary, requiring surgery in all cases, chemotherapy in most cases (except in setting of patients with VLRWT), and radiation therapy in higher-stage disease. Risk stratification, which includes molecular biomarkers, and in some cases response to initial chemotherapy, has allowed tailoring of therapy based on patients' risk of recurrence, ensuring that patients carrying poor prognostic factors receive the therapy they require for their best chance at survival. Further, through completed trials, we have also learned which patients have the most favorable prognoses and therefore can be spared additional and toxic therapy.

2.5.1 International Society of Paediatric Oncology

The SIOP approach to patients with suspected WT supports 4–6 weeks of chemotherapy prior to gross nephrectomy, as the use of neoadjuvant chemotherapy has been linked to a decreased risk of tumor spillage and lower postoperative stage [48]. For localized tumors, a 4-week treatment with weekly vincristine and biweekly dactinomycin is used. For metastatic tumors, the neoadjuvant treatment consists of 6 weeks of vincristine, dactinomycin, and doxorubicin. A radical nephroureterectomy is then performed with locoregional lymph node sampling. In exceptional cases, a partial nephrectomy may be considered. Following surgery, the tumor is classified according to stage and histologic subtype, based on local pathology assessment and central pathology review. A careful assessment of residual blastemal volume is performed since a higher volume of >10–20 ml is considered as an adverse prognostic factor. Patients are assigned to low-, intermediate-, and high-risk groups based on percentage of necrosis within the tumor and predominance of histological subtypes within the tumor (stromal, epithelial, and blastemal and focal/diffuse anaplasia) [48, 49]. Diffuse anaplasia and blastemal histology denote the patient as high-risk. The SIOP treatment approach and most recently reported outcomes according to stage and histology are summarized in Tables 2.3 and 2.4.

Table 2.3 SIOP 2001 treatment approach

Stage	Preoperative chemotherapy	Histology	Additional clinical/ biologic prognostic factors	Postoperative chemotherapy	Radiation therapy (XRT)
I	AV × 4 weeks	Low risk		None	None
		Intermediate risk	Postoperative tumor volume > 500 mL[a]	AV × 4 weeks	
		High risk		AVD × 27 weeks	
II	AV × 4 weeks	Low risk		AV × 27 weeks	None
		Intermediate risk	Postoperative tumor volume > 500 mL[a]	AV × 27 weeks vs. AVD × 27 weeks[b]	None
		High risk		CDCE × 34 weeks	25.2 Gy flank XRT for diffuse anaplasia
III	AV × 4 weeks	Low risk		AV × 27 weeks	None
		Intermediate risk	Postoperative tumor volume > 500 mL[a]	AV × 27 weeks vs. AVD × 27 weeks[b]	14.4 Gy flank XRT; 10.8 Gy boost for gross residual disease
		High risk		CDCE × 34 weeks	25.2 Gy flank XRT; 10.8 Gy boost for gross residual disease

(continued)

Table 2.3 (continued)

Stage	Preoperative chemotherapy	Histology	Additional clinical/ biologic prognostic factors	Postoperative chemotherapy	Radiation therapy (XRT)
IV	AVD × 6 weeks	Low risk	Lung nodule CR[c]	AVD × 27 weeks	Flank XRT for local stage III
			No lung CR[c]	CDCE × 34 weeks	15 Gy lung, flank XRT for local stage III
		Intermediate risk	Lung nodule CR[c]	AVD × 27 weeks	Flank XRT for local stage III
			No lung CR[c]	CDCE × 34 weeks	15 Gy lung; flank XRT for local stage III
		High risk	Lung nodule CR[c]	CDCE × 34 weeks	Flank XRT for local stage II/ III[d]
			No lung CR[c]	CDCE × 34 weeks	15 Gy lung; flank XRT for local stage II/ III[d]

SIOP international Society of Paediatric Oncology, *CR* complete response, *AV* dactinomycin/vincristine, *AVD* dactinomycin/vincristine/doxorubicin (cumulative doxorubicin dose, 250 mg/m^2 for stages I to III; 300 mg/m^2 for stage IV), *CDCE* cyclophosphamide/doxorubicin alternating with carboplatin/etoposide (cumulative doxorubicin dose, 300 mg/m^2 for stage IV)

[a]In Germany, tumor volume > 500 mL that was not epithelial or stromal predominant was designated as high-risk

[b]AV non-inferior to AVD according to results of randomized study SIOP 2001 [52]

[c]CR attained by chemotherapy and/or metastastectomy. Extrapulmonary metastases also underwent radiation, dose dependent on site

[d]Flank XRT was given for all high-risk stage III but was given only for stage II diffuse anaplasia and not stage II blastemal type. Metastasis in the presence of anaplastic primary tumor received radiation regardless of response

2.5.2 Children's Oncology Group

The COG approach to newly diagnosed WT calls for upfront nephrectomy followed by adjuvant chemotherapy. The goal of this methodology is to expedite diagnosis and allow for accurate histologic diagnosis. Also, lymph node involvement and tumor spillage can be accurately assessed [2]. Patients that have inoperable tumors or bilateral WT are exceptions and receive preoperative chemotherapy. COG histologic risk assignment is consolidated into three groups based on the lowest to highest risk: favorable histology, focal anaplasia, and diffuse anaplasia [2]. The presence of diffuse anaplasia dictates the need for additional chemotherapy agents (doxorubicin for stage I and doxorubicin, cyclophosphamide, etoposide, and carboplatin for stages II–IV) as well as flank radiation. Recent data from the COG AREN0321

Table 2.4 Outcomes reported on recent SIOP studies

Stage	Histology	Additional factors	5-year EFS	5-year OS	Comments
I	Intermediate risk and anaplasia		87% [50]	95% [50]	Results for group treated with only 4 weeks of chemo postsurgery
	Blastemal type		96% [51]	100% [51]	With 27 weeks of AVD
II/III	Intermediate risk		85% [52]	96% [52]	Results listed are for group treated without doxorubicin
	Blastemal type		79% [51]	84% [51]	With 34 weeks of CDCE
IV	Non-anaplastic	Pulmonary metastases only	77% [53]	87% [53]	—
	Anaplastic	Pulmonary metastases only	33% [53]	33% [53]	—

AVD dactinomycin/vincristine/doxorubicin, *CDCE* cyclophosphamide/doxorubicin alternating with carboplatin/etoposide

study showed that the vincristine/irinotecan combination was active in stage IV diffuse AHWT [54]. The COG treatment approach and outcomes based on the stage of disease are depicted in Tables 2.5 and 2.6.

2.5.3 Special Circumstances

2.5.3.1 Bilateral Wilms Tumor

Patients with bilateral WT, or stage V disease, are treated somewhat similarly within the COG and SIOP approaches. According to the recently completed COG study AREN0534, patients with bilateral WT underwent an initial 6–12 weeks of preoperative chemotherapy with vincristine, dactinomycin, and doxorubicin, with the hope of decreasing tumor size prior to bilateral nephron-sparing surgery [2]. Doxorubicin was added due to findings in an earlier study which showed decreased risk of relapse in patients with the added drug in comparison to those who received vincristine and dactinomycin alone (8% vs. 42%) [59]. Therapy after nephrectomy was based on tumor histology, similar to the SIOP histologic grading system. Patients with bilateral WT treated according to the most recent SIOP 2001 protocol were treated with vincristine and dactinomycin for the initial 6 weeks, with the addition of doxorubicin later on if warranted.

The local therapy should be discussed with expert surgeons in close collaboration with expert radiologists. Prolonged preoperative chemotherapy (up to 12 weeks) may be necessary in order to have maximal tumor shrinkage, thereby resulting in maximal nephron-sparing surgery. Not all renal masses contain WT but may contain nephrogenic rests that do not necessarily require surgery but merit adjuvant chemotherapy (up to 12–18 months).

Table 2.5 COG treatment approach (AREN0321, AREN0532, and AREN0533 trials)

Stage	Histology	Additional clinical/biologic factor	LOH 1p and 16q	Chemotherapy	Radiation therapy (XRT)
I	Favorable	Age < 2 years and tumor <550 g	Any	None	None
		Age ≥ 2 years or tumor ≥550 g	No	AV × 19 weeks	None
		Age ≥ 2 years or tumor ≥550 g	Yes	AVD × 25 weeks	None
	Focal anaplasia	Any	Any	AVD × 25 weeks	10.8 Gy flank
	Diffuse anaplasia	Any	Any	AVD × 25 weeks	10.8 Gy flank
II	Favorable		No	AV × 19 weeks	None
			Yes	AVD × 25 weeks	None
	Focal anaplasia		Any	AVD × 25 weeks	10.8 Gy flank
	Diffuse anaplasia		Any	VDCBE × 30 weeks	10.8 Gy flank
III	Favorable		No	AVD × 25 weeks	10.8 Gy flank/abdomen;
			Yes	VDACE × 31 weeks	10.8 Gy boost for gross disease
	Focal anaplasia		Any	AVD × 25 weeks	10.8 Gy flank/abdomen; 10.8 Gy boost for gross disease
	Diffuse anaplasia		Any	VDCBE × 30 weeks	20 Gy flank/abdomen; 10.8 Gy boost for gross disease
IV	Favorable	Lung nodule CR after week 6	No	AVD × 25 weeks	No lung XRT
		Lung nodule CR after week 6	Yes	VDACE × 31 weeks	12 Gy lung[a]
		No lung nodule CR after week 6	Any	VDACE × 31 weeks	12 Gy lung[a]
	Focal anaplasia	Any	Any	VDCBE × 30 weeks	12 Gy lung[a]
	Diffuse anaplasia	Any	Any	VDCBEI × 36 weeks[b]	12 Gy lung[a]

AV dactinomycin/vincristine, *AVD* dactinomycin/vincristine/doxorubicin (cumulative doxorubicin dose, 150 mg/m^2), *COG* Children's Oncology Group, *CR* complete response, *VDACE* vincristine/doxorubicin/dactinomycin/cyclophosphamide/etoposide (cumulative doxorubicin dose, 195 mg/m^2), *VDCBE* vincristine/doxorubicin/carboplatin/cyclophosphamide/etoposide, *VDCBEI* vincristine/doxorubicin/carboplatin/cyclophosphamide/etoposide/irinotecan (cumulative doxorubicin, dose 225 mg/m^2)

[a]Extrapulmonary metastatic sites also received radiation, dose dependent on site
[b]Patients received vincristine/irinotecan only if response was seen after 6 weeks of phase II window therapy

Table 2.6 Outcomes reported on recent NWTSG/COG studies

Stage	Histology	Additional clinical/ biologic factor	4-year EFS	4-year OS	Comments
I	Favorable	Age < 2 years and tumor <550 g	90% [46]	100% [46]	Nephrectomy only
		Age > 2 years OR tumor >550 g	94% [39]	98% [39]	Without LOH 1p
	Anaplasia	Focal or diffuse	100% [55]	100% [55]	With VDA/flank XRT
II	Favorable		86% [39]	98% [39]	Without LOH 1p
	Diffuse anaplasia		85% [55]	*	3-year EFS reported
III	Favorable		87% [39]	94% [39]	Without LOH 1p
	Diffuse anaplasia		74% [55]	*	3-year EFS reported
IV	Favorable	Lung metastases only; lung nodule CR after week 6	78% [56]	95% [56]	No lung XRT
		Lung metastases only; lung nodule IR after week 6	88% [57]	92% [57]	With VDACE/lung XRT 3-year EFS reported
		Extrapulmonary metastases	82% [58]	91% [58]	With VDACE/XRT
	Diffuse anaplasia		46% [54]	*	3-year EFS reported

EFS event-free survival, *OS* overall survival, *LOH* loss of heterozygosity, *VDA* vincristine/doxorubicin/dactinomycin, *VDACE* vincristine/doxorubicin/dactinomycin/cyclophosphamide/etoposide, *VDCBE* vincristine/doxorubicin/carboplatin/cyclophosphamide/etoposide, *XRT* radiation therapy, * Not reported, but EFS and OS for diffuse anaplastic Wilms tumor are nearly equivalent

Stage IV Disease

Patients with metastatic disease within the lungs, liver, or other distant sites at initial diagnosis are considered to have stage IV disease by both SIOP and COG staging systems. The lung is the most common metastatic site, affecting up to 20% of patients with WT. A challenge has been how to define pulmonary metastatic disease in the era of CT scans, which are more sensitive than chest x-rays but also prone to false-positive readings. Despite these limitations, CT scans have become a standard part of the staging workup in both COG and SIOP studies.

Patients with pulmonary nodules treated per SIOP protocols receive the initial three-drug regimen of vincristine, dactinomycin, and doxorubicin and then are reimaged after 6 weeks. If lung nodules have a complete response (CR) to chemotherapy or are completely resected, patients do not receive lung radiation (XRT). With this approach, approximately 80% of patients avoid lung irradiation [53].

In the past, per the NWTSG treatment approach, all patients with pulmonary metastasis were subjected to whole lung radiation. However, the recently completed trial AREN0533 omitted lung XRT for patients with FHWT and isolated lung metastasis whose lung nodules had CR to the initial 6 weeks of chemotherapy with vincristine, dactinomycin, and doxorubicin. A difference between the SIOP and COG studies is that on the COG studies, the nodules had to achieve CR with chemotherapy alone; if a patient was rendered with CR with surgical resection, lung XRT was given if there was viable tumor present in the resection sample. If the pulmonary nodules did not respond completely, biopsy was encouraged, and if WT was confirmed, patients underwent lung XRT, and cyclophosphamide and etoposide were added to the initial three-drug regimen. Patients with CR of lung nodules were able to avoid lung radiation without worsened event-free survival (EFS), and those who did not have complete response of nodules had improved EFS with addition of cyclophosphamide and etoposide [57].

Recurrent Disease

In the past, patients with recurrent WT had dismal outcomes [60]. Grundy et al. performed the first comprehensive review of patients with relapsed WT, including patients from NWTS-2 and NWTS-3. Unfavorable prognostic factors following patient relapse included time to relapse, with time to relapse between 0 and 6 months following the end of adjuvant chemotherapy associated with significantly decreased survival in comparison to relapse more than 6 months after treatment [61, 62]. More recent data from NWTS-5 showed that time to relapse no longer negatively affected outcome. Through collaboration between the COG and SIOP, a risk stratification schema has been created that takes into account not only the patients' histology but also previous treatment received [60].

During the past two decades, the discovery of new chemotherapy drugs has allowed for the improved survival of patients with recurrent WT. Results from NWTS-5 revealed that patients treated initially with vincristine and dactinomycin had an 80% survival rate after recurrence, whereas patients treated initially with three or more agents had a 50% survival rate after recurrence [63, 64]. Topotecan was found to have activity against relapsed WT, with an overall response rate of 48% in FHWT [65]. The role of high-dose therapy with autologous stem cell rescue has been the subject of considerable debate. Although a randomized clinical trial to assess the benefit of high-dose therapy has not been conducted, a meta-analysis of the available literature suggested that the benefit of high-dose therapy was restricted to patients who received more than four agents as part of their initial treatment [66].

2.6   Complications and Late Effects

Due to the outstanding survival rate in a large subset of patients with WT, some of the focus has shifted to diminishing the toxicities of treatment, especially those secondary to doxorubicin, alkylating agents, and radiation therapy. The cumulative risk for congestive heart failure at 20 years after the end of therapy was 4.4% in patients treated on NWTS protocols, with risk related to exposure to doxorubicin and lung radiation [67]. Those that do not develop heart failure can have milder yet significant cardiac dysfunction, and all who have history of exposure to doxorubicin ± lung radiation are followed closely with echocardiograms. The SIOP 2001 trial concluded that the use of doxorubicin does not improve outcome in standard-risk stage II and III WT, which will prevent cardiac sequelae in the future [52].

The risk of end-stage renal disease is quite low in patients with history of unilateral WT, affecting only 0.6%; however, in patients with history of bilateral WT, the frequency increases to 12%. Patients with underlying history of syndromes involving *WT1* such as WAGR or Denys-Drash have an even higher frequency of end-stage renal disease, at 34% and 74%, respectively [68].

Unfortunately, due to agents including doxorubicin, cyclophosphamide, and etoposide and radiation therapy, WT survivors are at increased risk for secondary malignancy. A cohort of 1256 WT survivors from the Childhood Cancer Survivor Study (CCSS) had a cumulative incidence of secondary malignant neoplasms of 3.0% at 25 years from the time of WT diagnosis [69]. Secondary cancers included acute leukemia, lymphoma, gastrointestinal and peritoneal tumors, brain tumors, sarcomas, melanoma, and breast cancer. A more recent report from the NWTS showed that the cumulative incidence of breast cancer at age 40 years in female survivors who received whole lung radiation was nearly 15% [70].

WT treatment can also be associated with infertility. Gonadal dysfunction with secondary infertility may result from exposure to high cumulative doses of cyclophosphamide ($>=9$ g/m^2), which is used for AHWT and some cases of higher-risk FHWT. In females, premature ovarian failure is a known complication of high cumulative doses of cyclophosphamide and radiation exposure. Flank radiation can also lead to development of hypertension, which may complicate pregnancy. Females who undergo flank radiation are more likely to have malposition, premature births, and low birth weight infants [67].

Hopefully, with the advent of future trials, improved understanding of important prognostic molecular markers, and discovery of novel, more targeted therapeutics with activity in WT, the sometimes substantial toxicities of current WT treatment can be evaded.

2.7 Future Directions

The excellent overall outcomes in patients with WT are the result of successive collaborative clinical trials. Despite the fact that over 90% of patients survive, there is still a significant subset of patients that are at risk for unsatisfactory outcomes, especially following relapse. Unfortunately, we are reaching the limits of tolerability and efficacy with known chemotherapy agents and radiation therapy, creating a need for novel and more targeted treatments. In those who do survive, there is potential for the development of chronic health issues that can significantly affect quality of life. As outcomes have improved and biomarkers have divided patients into relatively small risk groups, there has been an increased need for partnership between COG and SIOP in order to conduct clinical trials of sufficient size to draw meaningful conclusions. There is continued need to focus on the paradox of improving outcomes while lessening the toxicities of our treatment regimens.

References

1. Dome JS, Perlman EJ, Graf N. Risk stratification for Wilms tumor: current approach and future directions. Am Soc Clin Oncol Educ Book. 2014:215–23. https://doi.org/10.14694/EdBook_AM.2014.34.215.
2. Dome JS, Graf N, Geller JI, et al. Advances in Wilms Tumor Treatment and Biology: Progress Through International Collaboration. J Clin Oncol. 2015;33(27):2999–3007.
3. Chu A, Heck J, Ribeiro KB, Brennan P, Boffeta P, Buffler P, Hung RJ. Wilms' tumour: a systematic review of risk factors and meta-analysis. Paediatr Perinat Epidemiol. 2010;24:449–69.
4. Howlader N, Noone AM, Krapcho M, et al. SEER Cancer Statistics Review, 1975–2014. Bethesda, MD., https://seer.cancer.gov/csr/1975_2014/, based on November 2016 SEER data submission, posted to the SEER web site, April: National Cancer Institute; 2017.
5. Ali A, Diaz R, Shu HK, Paulino AC, Esiashvil N. A Surveillance, Epidemiology, and End Results (SEER) Program Comparison of Adult and Pediatric Wilms' Tumor. Cancer. 2012;118:2541–51.
6. Wilms M. Die Mischgeschwilste. Leipzig: A Georgi Leipzig; 1899. p. 1–90.
7. Szychot E, Apps J, Pritchard-Jones K. Wilms' tumor biology, diagnosis and treatment. Transl Pediatr. 2014;3(1):12–24.
8. Rivera MN, Haber DA. Wilms' tumour: connecting tumorigenesis and organ development in the kidney. Nat Rev Cancer. 2005;5(9):699–712.
9. Scott RH, Stiller CA, Walker L, et al. Syndromes and constitutional chromosomal abnormalities associated with Wilms tumour. J Med Genet. 2006;43(9):705–15.
10. Breslow NE, Olson J, Moksness J, et al. Familial Wilms' tumor: A descriptive study. Med Pediatr Oncol. 1996;27:398–403.
11. Doumoucel S, Gauthier-Villars M, Stoppa-Lyonnet D, et al. Malformations, Genetic Abnormalities, and Wilms Tumor. Pediatr Blood Cancer. 2014;61:140–4.
12. Royer-Pokora B, Beier M, Henzler M, et al. Twenty-four new cases of WT-1 germ line mutations and review of the literature: genotype phenotype correlations for Wilms tumor development. Am J Med Genet Part A. 2004;127A:249–57.
13. Scott RH, Douglas J, Baskcomb L, et al. Constitutional 11p15 abnormalities, including heritable imprinting center mutations, cause nonsyndromic Wilms tumor. Nat Genet. 2008;40(11):1329–34.
14. Rump P, Zeegers MPA, van Essen AJ, et al. Tumor risk in Beckwith-Wiedemann Syndrome: A review and meta-analysis. Am J Med Genet A. 2005;136(1):95–104.
15. Kreidberg JA, Sariola H, Loring JM, et al. WT-1 is required for early kidney development. Cell. 1993;74(4):679–91.
16. Koesters R, Ridder R, Kopp-Schneider A, et al. Mutational Activation of the β-Catenin Proto-Oncogene Is a Common Event in the Development of Wilms' Tumors. Cancer Res. 1999;59(16):3880–2.
17. Maiti S, Alam R, Amos CI, et al. Frequent association of beta-catenin and WT1 mutations in Wilms tumors. Cancer Res. 2000;60(22):6288–92.
18. Fukuzawa R, Anaka MR, Weeks RJ, Morison IM, Reeve AE. Canonical WNT signaling determines lineage specificity in Wilms tumour. Oncogene. 2009;28(8):1063–75.
19. Ruteshouser EC, Robinson SM, Huff V. Wilms tumor genetics: mutations in WT1, WTX, and CTNNB1 account for only about one-third of tumors. Genes Chromosomes Cancer. 2009;47(6):461–70.
20. Rivera MN, Kim WJ, Wells J, et al. An X chromosome gene, WTX, is commonly inactivated in Wilms tumor. Science. 2007;315(5812):642–5.
21. Wegert J, Ishaque N, Vardapour R, et al. Mutations in the SIX1/2 pathway and the DROSHA/DGCR8 miRNA microprocessor complex underlie high-risk blastemal type Wilms tumors. Cancer Cell. 2015;27(2):298–311.
22. Walz AL, Ooms AH, Gadd S, et al. Recurrent DGCR8, DROSHA, and SIX Homeodomain Mutations in Favorable Histology Wilms Tumors. Cancer Cell. 2015;27(2):286–97.

23. Rakheja D, Chen KS, Liu Y, et al. Somatic mutations in DROSHA and DICER1 impair microRNA biogenesis through distinct mechanisms in Wilms tumors. Nat Commun. 2014;2:4802.
24. Torrezan GT, Ferreira EN, Nakahata AM, et al. Recurrent somatic mutation in DROSHA induces microRNA profile changes in Wilms tumour. Nat Commun. 2014;5:4039.
25. Perlman EJ, Gadd S, Arold ST, et al. MLLT1 YEATS domain mutations in clinically distinctive Favourable histology Wilms tumours. Nat Commun. 2015;6:10013.
26. Irtan S, Ehrlich P, Pritchard-Jones K. Wilms tumor: 'State-of-the-art' update, 2016. Semin Pediatr Surg. 2016;25(5):250–6.
27. Malkan AD, Loh A, Bahrami A, et al. An Approach to Renal Masses in Pediatrics. Pediatrics. 2015;135(1):142–58.
28. Smets AMJB, van Tinteren H, Bergeron C, et al. The contribution of chest CT-scan at diagnosis in children with unilateral Wilms' tumour. Results of the SIOP 2001 study. Eur J Cancer. 2012;48(7):1060–5.
29. Ehrlich PF, Hamilton TE, Grundy P, et al. The value of surgery in directing therapy for patients with Wilms' tumor with pulmonary disease. A report from the National Wilms' Tumor Study Group/National Wilms' Tumor Study 5. J Pediatr Surg. 2006;41(1):162–7.
30. Wilimas JA, Kaste SC, Kauffman WM, et al. Use of chest computed tomography in the staging of pediatric Wilms' tumor: interobserver variability and prognostic significance. J Clin Oncol. 1997;15(7):2631–5.
31. Owens CM, Veys PA, Pritchard J, et al. Role of chest computed tomography at diagnosis in the management of Wilms' tumor: a study by the United Kingdom Children's Cancer Study Group. J Clin Oncol. 2002;20(12):2768–73.
32. Grundy PE, Green DM, Dirks AC, et al. Clinical Significance of Pulmonary Nodules Detected by CT and Not CXR Patients Treated for Favorable Histology Wilms Tumor on National Wilms Tumor Studies-4 and -5: A Report from the Children's Oncology Group. Pediatr Blood Cancer. 2012;59:631–5.
33. Coppes MJ, Zandvoort SW, Sparling CR, et al. Acquired von Willebrand disease in Wilms' tumor patients. J Clin Oncol. 1992;10(3):422–7.
34. Beckwith JB. Nephrogenic Rest and the Pathogenesis of Wilms Tumor: Developmental and Clinical Considerations. Am J Med Genet. 1998;79:268–79.
35. Spreafico F, Terenziani M, Fossati-Blanni F, et al. Revised SIOP working classification of renal tumors of childhood. Med Pediatr Oncol. 2003;41(1):102.
36. Geller JI. Current standards of care and future directions for "high-risk" pediatric renal tumors: Anaplastic Wilms tumor and Rhabdoid tumor. Urol Oncol. 2016;34:50–6.
37. Maschietto M, Williams RD, Chagtai T, et al. TP53 Mutational Status Is a Potential Marker for Risk Stratification in Wilms Tumour with Diffuse Anaplasia. PLoS One. 2014;9(10):1–8.
38. Ooms AH, Gadd S, Gerhard DS, et al. Significance of TP53 Mutation in Wilms Tumors with Diffuse Anaplasia: A Report from the Children's Oncology Group. Clin Cancer Res. 2016;22(22):5582–91.
39. Grundy PE, Breslow NE, Li S, et al. Loss of Heterozygosity for Chromosomes 1p and 16q Is an Adverse Prognostic Factor in Favorable-Histology Wilms Tumor: A Report From the National Wilms Tumor Study Group. J Clin Oncol. 2005;23(29):7312–21.
40. Chagtai T, Zill C, Dainese L, et al. Gain of 1q As a Prognostic Biomarker in Wilms Tumors (WTs) Treated with Preoperative Chemotherapy in the International Society of Paediatric Oncology (SIOP) WT 2001 Trial: A SIOP Renal Tumour Biology Consortium Study. J Clin Oncol. 2016;34(26):3196–203.
41. Gratias EJ, Dome JS, Jennings LJ, et al. Association of Chromosome 1q Gain With Inferior Survival in Favorable-Histology Wilms Tumor: A Report From the Children's Oncology Group. J Clin Oncol. 2016;34(26):3189–94.
42. Gratias EJ, Jennings LJ, Anderson JR, et al. Gain of 1q is associated with inferior event-free and overall survival in patients with favorable histology Wilms tumor: a report from the Children's Oncology Group. Cancer. 2013;119(21):3887–94.

43. Pritchard-Jones K, Kelsey A, Imeson VJ, et al. Older Age Is an Adverse Prognostic Factor in Stage I Favorable Histology Wilms' Tumor Treated With Vincristine Monochemotherapy: A Study by the United Kingdom Children's Cancer Study Group, Wilm's Tumor Working Group. J Clin Oncol. 2003;21:3269–75.
44. Green DM, Breslow NE, Beckwith B, et al. Treatment Outcomes in Patients Less than 2 Years of Age with Small, Stage I, Favorable-Histology Wilms' Tumors: A Report from the National Wilms' Tumor Study. J Clin Oncol. 1993;11:91–5.
45. Green DM, Breslow NE, Beckwith B, et al. Treatment With Nephrectomy Only for Small, Stage I/Favorable Histology Wilms' Tumor: A Report From the National Wilms' Tumor Study Group. J Clin Oncol. 2001;19:3719–24.
46. Fernandez CV, Perlman EJ, Mullen EA, et al. Clinical Outcome and Biological Predictors of Relapse After Nephrectomy Only for Very Low-risk Wilms Tumor: A Report From Children's Oncology Group AREN0532. Ann Surg. 2017;265(4):835–40.
47. Perlman EJ, Grundy PE, Anderson JR, et al. WT1 Mutation and 11p15 Loss of Heterozygosity Predict Relapse in Very Low-Risk Wilms Tumors Treated with Surgery Alone: A Children's Oncology Group Study. J Clin Oncol. 2010;29:698–703.
48. Graf N, Tournade MF, de Kraker J. The role of preoperative chemotherapy in the management of Wilms' tumor: The SIOP studies. Urol Clin North Am. 2000;27:443–54.
49. Vujanic GM, Sandstedt B, Harms D, et al. Revised International Society of Paediatric Oncology (SIOP) working classification of renal tumors of childhood. Med Pediatr Oncol. 2002;38:79–82.
50. de Kraker J, Graf N, van Tinteren H, et al. Reduction of postoperative chemotherapy in children with stage I intermediate-risk and anaplastic Wilms' tumor (SIOP 93-01 trial): a randomized controlled trial. Lancet. 2004;364(9441):1229–35.
51. van den Heuvel-Eibrink MM, van Tinteren H, Bergeron C, et al. Outcome of localized blastemal-type Wilms tumour patients treated according to intensified treatment in the SIOP WT 2001 protocol, a report of the SIOP Renal Tumour Study Group (SIOP-RTSG). Eur J Cancer. 2015;51:498–506.
52. Pritchard-Jones K, Bergeron C, Camargo B, et al. Omission of doxorubicin from treatment of II-III, intermediate-risk Wilms' tumour (SIOP WT-2001): an open-label, non-inferiority randomized controlled trial. Lancet. 2015;386(999):1156–64.
53. Verschuur A, Van Tinteren H, Graf N, et al. Treatment of pulmonary metastases in children with stage IV nephroblastoma with risk-based use of pulmonary radiotherapy. J Clin Oncol. 2012;30:3533–9.
54. Daw NC, Anderson JR, Hoffer FA, et al. A phase 2 study of vincristine and irinotecan in metastatic diffuse anaplastic Wilms tumor: Results from the Children's Oncology Group AREN0321 study. J Clin Oncol. 2014;32(15s):1032.
55. Daw NC, Anderson JR, Kalapurakal JA, et al. Treatment of stage II-IV diffuse anaplastic Wilms tumor: Results from the Children's Oncology Group AREN0321 study. Presented at the 46th congress of the international society of paediatric oncology, 22–25 Oct 2014, Toronto, ON.
56. Dix DB, Gratias EJ, Seibel N, et al. Omission of lung radiation in patients with stage IV favorable histology Wilms Tumor (FHWT) showing complete lung nodule response after chemotherapy: A report from Children's Oncology Group study AREN0533. J Clin Oncol. 2015;33(15):10011.
57. Dix DB, Gratias EJ, Seibel N, et al. Treatment of stage IV favorable histology Wilms tumor with incomplete lung metastasis response after chemotherapy: A report from the Children's Oncology Group study AREN0533. J Clin Oncol. 2014;32(5s):10001.
58. Dix DB, Gratias E, Seibel NI, et al. Treatment of stage IV favorable histology wilms tumor with extra-pulmonary metastases: a report from Children's Oncology Group Study AREN0533. Presented at the 48th congress of the international society of paediatric oncology, 19–22 Oct 2016, Dublin.
59. Paulino AC, Wilimas J, Marina N, et al. Local control in synchronous bilateral Wilms tumor. Int J Radiat Oncol Biol Phys. 1996;36:541–8.

60. Spreafico F, Pritchard Jones K, Malogolowkin MH, et al. Treatment of relapsed Wilms tumors: lessons learned. Expert Rev Anticancer Ther. 2009;9(12):1807–15.
61. D'Angio GJ, Evans A, Breslow N, et al. The treatment of Wilms' tumor: results of the Second National Wilms' Tumor Study. Cancer. 1981;47(9):2302–11.
62. D'Angio GJ, Evans AE, Breslow N, et al. The treatment of Wilms' tumor: Results of the national Wilms' tumor study. Cancer. 1976;38(2):633–46.
63. Green DM, Cotton CA, Malogolowkin M, et al. Treatment of Wilms tumor relapsing after initial treatment with vincristine, actinomycin D: a report from the National Wilms Tumor Study Group. Pediatr Blood Cancer. 2007;48(5):493–9.
64. Malogolowkin M, Math CACM, Green DM, et al. Treatment of Wilms tumor relapsing after initial treatment with vincristine, actinomycin D, and doxorubicin. A report from the National Wilms Tumor Study Group. Pediatr Blood Cancer. 2008;50(2):236–41.
65. Metzger ML, Stewart CF, Freeman BB, et al. Topotecan Is Active Against Wilms' Tumor: Results of a Multi-Institutional Phase II Study. J Clin Oncol. 2007;25(21):3130–6.
66. Ha TC, Spreafico F, Graf N, et al. An international strategy to determine the role of high dose therapy in recurrent Wilms' tumour. Eur J Cancer. 2013;49(2):194–210.
67. Wright KD, Green DM, Daw NC. Late Effects of Treatment for Wilms Tumor. Pediatr Hematol Oncol. 2009;26(6):407–13.
68. Breslow NE, Grigoriev YA, Peterson SM, et al. End Stage Renal Disease in Patients With Wilms Tumor: Results from the National Wilms Tumor Study Group and the U.S. Renal Data System. J Urol. 2005;174(5):1972–5.
69. Breslow NE, Lange JM, Friedman DL, et al. Secondary Malignant Neoplasms following Wilms Tumor: An International Collaborative Study. Int J Cancer. 2010;127(3):657–66.
70. Lange JM, Takashima JR, Peterson SM, et al. Breast cancer in female survivors of Wilms tumor: a report from the national Wilms tumor late effects study. Cancer. 2014;120(23):3722–30.

Ryan D. Bitar and Najat C. Daw

Renal cell carcinoma (RCC) is a group of malignancies arising from the epithelium of the renal tubules [1]. Renal tumors account for 3–4% of all malignant tumors in adults, and 80–90% of these are RCCs [2]. The mean age at diagnosis is 68 years in men and 71 years in women [2]. While RCC is the most prevalent renal tumor in adults, it is extremely rare in children. Data from the National Program of Cancer Registries and Surveillance, Epidemiology, and End Results (SEER) statewide registries from 2001 to 2009 showed the incidence rate of renal tumors in children and adolescents (ages 0–19 years) in the United States to be 6.64% and that of renal carcinomas 0.61% [3]. Whereas nephroblastoma, also known as Wilms tumor, accounts for approximately 90% of Paediatric renal tumors, renal carcinomas account for less than 10% of them [3]. RCCs are more common than clear-cell sarcoma of the kidney or rhabdoid tumors of the kidney. Due to the plethora of adult renal cases, inferences from the nature of adult disease were projected on the Paediatric disease; however, major biological differences between adult and Paediatric renal carcinoma exist. Indeed, Paediatric RCC is biologically unique when compared to adult RCC.

3.1   Epidemiology

Little is known about the epidemiology of RCC in children due to the rarity of this disease. The annual incidence rate is approximately 4 cases per one million children [4]. Although Wilms tumor is the predominant renal tumor in childhood, it is rare

R. D. Bitar
The University of Texas Health Science Center at San Antonio, San Antonio, TX, USA

N. C. Daw (✉)
Department of Paediatrics, The University of Texas MD Anderson Cancer Center,
Houston, TX, USA
e-mail: NDaw@mdanderson.org

© Springer Nature Switzerland AG 2019
G. G. Malouf, N. M. Tannir (eds.), *Rare Kidney Tumors*,
https://doi.org/10.1007/978-3-319-96989-3_3

past early childhood, and RCC is the most prevalent renal malignancy during the second decade of life. In the older age group of adolescents (aged 15–19 years), approximately two-thirds of renal malignancies are RCC [5, 6]. In a report from the Children's Oncology Group (COG), the median age at diagnosis of 120 patients with unilateral RCC was 12.9 years (range, 1.9–22.1 years) [7].

Based on epidemiological adult studies, RCC has a male predominance, and its incidence rates in the United States are highest among African Americans and lowest among Asian/Pacific Islanders [8]. The incidence rates for white Hispanics in the United States are much higher than rates reported in Latin America, suggesting the potential role of environmental factors [8]. Smoking, obesity, and hypertension increase the risk of RCC, and a reduction in blood pressure lowers the risk [8–10]. Data on 43 cases of RCC in patients younger than 21 years from the California Cancer Registry showed that the overall annual age-adjusted incidence was 0.01/100,000, with the tumor more common in non-Hispanic blacks (0.03/100,000) when compared to non-Hispanic whites (0.01/100,000), Hispanics (<0.01/100,000), and non-Hispanic Asians/Pacific Islanders (<0.01/100,000) [11]. This study found more cases of RCC in females (58%) compared to males (42%); however, the COG study of 120 patients and the German study of 49 patients found that Paediatric RCC appears to have no sex predilection [7, 12]. The rates of renal carcinoma are increasing among children and adolescents; the increased rates of obesity among adolescents might explain increases in renal carcinomas observed overall and among those aged 15 to 19 years [3].

3.2   Genetics

RCC occurs in both sporadic and familial forms. Familial RCC syndromes, although rare, provide an invaluable model to study the molecular mechanisms of renal carcinogenesis. Many causative oncogenes and tumor suppressor genes have been identified, and it is now possible to identify the affected individuals and carriers by genetic testing [13]. Several genetic disorders are associated with a predisposition to RCC (Table 3.1).

Table 3.1 Genetic disorders associated with RCC

Disorder	Clinical manifestations	Mode of inheritance	Gene
Von Hippel–Lindau	Hemangioblastomas, retinal angiomas, RCC, pheochromocytomas, and pancreatic neuroendocrine tumors	Autosomal dominant	*VHL* gene
Tuberous sclerosis	Seizures, mental retardation, multiple hamartomas, renal angiomyolipomas, clear-cell RCC	Autosomal dominant	*TSC1* or *TSC2* genes
Birt–Hogg–Dubé syndrome	Hair follicle hamartomas, spontaneous pneumothorax, and susceptibility to hybrid oncocytoma/chromophobe RCC	Autosomal dominant	*FLCN* gene
Hereditary leiomyomatosis and renal cell cancer	Cutaneous leiomyomas, early-onset multiple uterine leiomyomas, and type 2 papillary RCC	Autosomal dominant	*FH* gene

Von Hippel-Lindau (VHL) syndrome is an autosomal dominantly inherited condition, caused by mutations or deletions in the *VHL* gene, a tumor suppressor gene which regulates the level of hypoxia-inducible factor family of transcription factors [14, 15]. This syndrome is characterized by central nervous system hemangioblastomas, retinal angiomas, and the development of RCC, usually of the clear-cell type, pheochromocytomas, and pancreatic neuroendocrine tumors. VHL-associated RCCs usually occur in adulthood and rarely in childhood.

Tuberous sclerosis is a multisystem autosomal dominant disorder caused by mutations in the *TSC1* and *TSC2* genes, which encode key regulators in the mammalian target of rapamycin (mTOR) pathway [16]. It is characterized by seizures, mental retardation, multiple hamartomas, renal angiomyolipomas, and the development of the clear-cell type of RCC.

Birt-Hogg-Dubé syndrome is an autosomal dominant genetic disorder caused by mutations in the tumor suppressor gene, *FLCN*, which interferes with the ability of folliculin to restrain cell growth and division [14, 17]. This syndrome is characterized by hair follicle hamartomas, spontaneous pneumothorax, and susceptibility to hybrid oncocytoma/chromophobe RCC [17].

Hereditary leiomyomatosis and renal cell cancer (HLRCC) is an autosomal dominant condition in which susceptible individuals are at risk for the development of cutaneous leiomyomas, early-onset multiple uterine leiomyomas, and an aggressive form of type 2 papillary renal cell cancer. HLRCC is caused by germline mutations in the tricarboxylic acid (Krebs) cycle, fumarate hydratase (*FH*) gene [18, 19].

Germline mutations in the *MET* proto-oncogene were identified in affected members of families with hereditary papillary renal carcinoma and in a subset of sporadic papillary renal carcinomas [20]. The pattern of inheritance of hereditary papillary renal carcinoma is consistent with autosomal dominant transmission with reduced penetrance. Correlation of papillary RCC type with *c-met* mutations has shown all of the tumors with this mutation to be type 1; however, not all type 1 papillary RCCs had c-met mutations [21].

Renal medullary carcinoma is seen typically in young patients with sickle cell trait, possibly due to the chronic ischemic damage of the epithelium of the renal papillae related to sickled erythrocytes [22].

3.3 Pathology

The 2016 World Health Organization (WHO) renal tumor classification lists several different subtypes of RCC; however, many of these tumor types are seldom seen in children [23]. The most common subtypes seen preferentially in children are the translocation-associated tumors, papillary RCC, renal medullary carcinoma, and oncocytic RCC following neuroblastoma [24]. Importantly, 21% of Paediatric RCC cannot be readily classified due to atypical features. The clear-cell RCC is the most common subtype seen in adults, accounting for 75% of the cases [25]. However, true adult-type clear-cell RCC associated with 3p25 (VHL locus) abnormalities rarely occurs in children [12, 24, 26]. Conventional clear-cell RCC was thought to comprise of 6–20% of Paediatric RCCs; however, many cases appear histologically atypical or have morphologic features of the translocation subtype [24].

The translocation-type RCC, the most common subtype in children, accounted for 46.7% of the 120 Paediatric RCCs that were centrally reviewed through the COG classification and biology study [7]. This subtype is characterized by translocations most frequently involving the TFE3 gene on chromosome Xp11.2 or the TFEB gene on chromosome 6p21 [27–29]. TFE3 and TFEB are members of the MiTF/TFE family, a subgroup of basic helix-loop-helix leucine zipper transcription factors. The most common fusion partners include the ASPL gene (17q25) and the PRCC gene (1q21). The histologic spectrum of translocation RCC is quite broad, and the histologic features of translocation-type RCC do not greatly differ based on fusion partners. The cells often contain abundant clear to variably eosinophilic cytoplasm and possess distinct cell borders separated by thin fibrovascular septa [24]. The combination of TFE3 immunohistochemistry and fluorescence in situ hybridization is an accurate and cost-effective approach for diagnosis of Xp11 translocation RCC [30].

In the COG classification and biology study, RCC not otherwise specified occurred in 20.8% of cases, papillary in 16.7%, renal medullary carcinoma in 10.8%, chromophobe in 3.3%, oncocytoma in 0.8%, and clear cell in 0.8%. Two types of papillary RCC are identified based on their histologic characteristics: Type 1 tumors are composed of cuboidal cells with scanty pale cytoplasm arranged in a single layer on the basement membrane of papillary cores, whereas type 2 tumors contain pseudostratified cells with higher nuclear grade and typically more eosinophilic cytoplasm [24]. The two types have distinct molecular and cytogenetic profiles in adults [31]. Chromosomal gains, particularly of 7p and 17p, are more frequently seen in type 1 papillary RCC, whereas in type 2 papillary RCC, there is a wide variety of chromosomal region gains and losses [31]. The histologic type is relevant to patient outcome; type 1 papillary RCC is clinically less aggressive than type 2, and sporadic type 1 papillary RCC is often indolent and less likely to metastasize [31, 32].

Renal medullary carcinomas are usually composed of high-grade epithelial cells with acidophilic cytoplasm, arranged in a tubular, often cribriform architecture; they occasionally are solid or sarcomatoid [33]. Distinct features of this subtype include desmoplasia and an acute inflammatory infiltrate [24]. The cytology may resemble rhabdoid tumors, and renal medullary carcinoma may also show loss of nuclear INI-1 protein. These tumors tend to be poorly circumscribed arising centrally in the renal medulla; hemorrhage and necrosis are common findings [22]. Renal medullary carcinoma afflicts young individuals with sickle cell hemoglobinopathy [33]. The strong vascular endothelial growth factor and hypoxia-inducible factor expression and positivity for TP53 in these tumors suggest that chronic medullary hypoxia secondary to hemoglobinopathy may be involved in the pathogenesis of renal medullary carcinomas [33].

Another distinct yet extremely rare subtype of RCCs is neuroblastoma-associated RCC. It can be single, bilateral, or multifocal and may develop in the early years of follow-up after neuroblastoma in children or, more commonly, years later in young adults [34, 35]. This ambiguous and heterogeneous subtype has variable morphology including papillary morphology, clear-cell morphology, anaplastic morphology, and oncocytoid or eosinophilic features [34]. The reason neuroblastoma survivors are prone to developing RCC is unknown; however, genetic predisposition, previous chemotherapy, and radiation treatment likely play a role [34]. RCC with Xp11.2 translocation was reported after treatment for neuroblastoma [36].

Tumor grading is a diagnostic factor used to assess the aggressiveness of the disease. The Fuhrman system was the most frequently used grading system in RCC, but grading systems relying solely on nucleolar prominence have shown a stronger association with patient outcome than those relying on Fuhrman grade for clear-cell and papillary RCC. The WHO recommends using the new four-tiered WHO/ International Society of Urological Pathology grading system [23, 37], which has been validated for clear-cell RCC and papillary RCC, but not for other less common tumor types. This grading system, as outlined in the WHO 2016 tumor classification report [23], describes whether tumor nucleoli are absent or inconspicuous and basophilic at ×400 magnification (grade 1), conspicuous and eosinophilic at ×400 magnification (grade 2) or ×100 magnification (grade 3), and whether there is extreme nuclear pleomorphism, multinucleate giant cells, and/or rhabdoid and/or sarcomatoid differentiation (grade 4) [37]. The grading system that will be most meaningful in Paediatric tumors is currently unknown [24].

3.4   Clinical Presentation

Children with RCC are typically older than children with Wilms tumor; the median age at diagnosis of RCC is 10–13 years [7, 12, 38, 39]. The most common symptoms are hematuria, abdominal or flank pain, and an abdominal mass. However, Paediatric RCC seldom presents with a collective triad of these symptoms [38]. In fact, an abdominal mass is typically not evident from physical examination, as RCC typically does not reach the size of most Wilms tumors. Other rare urogenital symptoms include dysuria and urinary retention [12]. Other presenting features include systemic symptoms such as fever, anemia, malaise, and weight loss [12, 40]. Unlike Wilms tumor, RCC is rarely asymptomatic and discovered incidentally on imaging studies (12–15% of cases) [12, 41]. Table 3.2 summarizes some of the differences between Paediatric RCC and Wilms tumor.

Clinically, RCC behaves somewhat differently in children than in adults. Children usually present with signs and symptoms related to their primary tumor (mass, pain, hematuria), whereas adults often present with signs and symptoms of metastatic disease or paraneoplastic phenomena [42]. Paraneoplastic syndromes in adults include hypercalcemia (pseudohyperparathyroidism), erythrocytosis, hypertension (erythropoietin), and gynecomastia (gonadotropin or prolactin). However, these syndromes are infrequently documented in children with RCC [43, 44]. Polycythemia, hypertension, fever, and weight loss have been reported in children [43]. Multifocality in Paediatric RCC is unusual and when present may point toward an underlying syndrome, such as tuberous sclerosis or von Hippel–Lindau disease. Bilateral involvement with RCC is extremely rare in children; the neuroblastoma-associated oncocytic RCCs are often multifocal or bilateral [7, 35, 38].

Table 3.2 Clinical characteristics of Paediatric RCC vs. Wilms tumor

Characteristic	RCC	Wilms tumor
Median age at presentation	10–13 years	3 years
Symptoms at presentation	Hematuria, abdominal or flank pain	Often asymptomatic and discovered incidentally
Sites of metastasis	Lymph nodes Lung, liver, and bone	Lymph nodes Lung
Diagnosis	Made by biopsy	Made by imaging studies and confirmed by histology at the time of nephrectomy
Treatment	Surgery is primary treatment Not sensitive to chemotherapy or radiotherapy	Treated by surgery Sensitive to chemotherapy and radiotherapy
Prognosis	Poor if unresectable disease or metastatic disease	Excellent except for advanced stage diffuse anaplastic Wilms tumor

3.5   Diagnosis

The diagnostic workup for children with RCC includes obtaining history, physical examination, abdominal ultrasound, and computerized tomography (CT) scan of the chest and abdomen. While ultrasound can reveal the presence of a renal mass, CT scan typically reveals a large, heterogeneous, solid mass with either well-circumscribed or poorly defined borders [45]. Intravenous enhancement of the tumor is usually less than the adjacent normal parenchyma. RCC tends to be smaller than WT and invades tissues locally with distortion of normal renal architecture and formation of a pseudocapsule that contains foci of calcification. Regional lymphadenopathy and vascular invasion are commonly seen [46]. In addition, cross-sectional imaging of the chest and abdomen should be taken in order to detect lung metastasis, enlarged retroperitoneal lymph nodes, and other metastatic sites [47]. Bone scintigraphy and imaging of the brain are considered only in symptomatic patients. The COG study found that 40% of the Paediatric patients with RCC present with either lymphatic or hematogenous spread; 19% have distant metastasis [7]. The most common site of metastases at the time of diagnosis is the lung, followed by the liver and bone.

Biopsy is necessary to establish the diagnosis. While the diagnosis of Wilms tumor is usually made by imaging studies and confirmed by histology at the time of nephrectomy, a core needle biopsy obtained via a posterior approach (to limit contamination of the peritoneal cavity) should be performed in patients with renal tumors who are older than 10 years, those with signs of infection or inflammation, or those with imaging findings such as significant adenopathy, no renal parenchyma seen, or intratumoral calcification. Although needle biopsy may present potential risks (bleeding, tumor seeding, arteriovenous fistula, infection, and pneumothorax along the needle tract) [48], improvements in techniques and physician expertise have momentously decreased the chance of complications and increased the diagnostic accuracy of percutaneous needle core biopsy. Guidance by ultrasonography or CT allows better needle localization and tumor visualization [49]. Additionally, lymph node evaluation is crucial in the workup of patients with RCC.

3.6 Staging

The staging system for RCC uses the American Joint Committee on Cancer TNM classification, which categorizes cases based on tumor size, local tumor extent, and presence or absence of metastasis. Stage grouping consists of four stages and takes into account (1) the tumor greatest dimension (7 cm or less vs. greater than 7 cm); (2) whether the tumor is limited to the kidney, extends into the renal veins or vena cava, or directly invades the adrenal gland, perinephric tissues, or Gerota's fascia; (3) regional lymph node metastasis; and (4) distant metastasis [1]. Children and adolescents with RCC present with more advanced disease than patients aged 21 to 30 years [4]. Of 304 children, ages 0 to 17 years, with RCC registered in the National Cancer Database, 39% had stage I disease, 16% stage II, 33% stage III, and 12% stage IV [39]. In terms of histologic subtype, over 90% of patients with renal medullary carcinoma present with stage IV disease, 63% of patients with translocation-type RCC present with advanced disease (stage III or IV), and 39% of patients without translocation-type RCC or renal medullary carcinoma present with advanced disease (stage III or IV) [7].

3.7 Treatment

The primary treatment of RCC is surgery, regardless of subtype. More than 80% of children with RCC undergo some type of resection. Radical nephrectomy, the most common initial surgical procedure, is performed in approximately 70% of the cases, and partial nephrectomy in approximately 15% [7, 39]. Patients with localized disease (stage I and II) could be cured by nephrectomy alone [14, 38]. Patients who do not undergo resection have a lower 5-year survival (20%) than those who undergo complete nephrectomy (79%) or partial nephrectomy (100%) [39]. Although partial nephrectomy is generally recommended for adult patients with tumors less than 7 cm, the limited information on partial nephrectomy in children suggest that children with tumors 4 cm or less and lower stage may undergo partial nephrectomy with excellent outcome [39]. Because of the importance of complete tumor resection and the lack of effective medical therapies, partial nephrectomy should be reserved for selected cases where complete resection with negative margins can be obtained [7]. The COG guidelines emphasize the importance of lymph node sampling from the renal hilum and the paracaval or para-aortic areas and excision of involved or suspicious lymph nodes at the time of surgery for accurate staging of renal tumors [7]. However, the need for radical lymph node dissection in management of Paediatric RCC, as in adult RCC, remains unclear [7, 14]. A systematic review of the literature found that local lymph node involvement does not predict poor outcome in Paediatric RCC and did not support the necessity of lymph node dissection [40]; however, other studies noted that regional lymph node involvement was associated with worse survival in children and recommended lymph node dissection for node-positive patients [39, 50].

Besides surgery, there is no established optimal treatment for childhood RCC regardless of subtype. Neither chemotherapy nor radiation therapy has demonstrated significant activity in adult or Paediatric patients with metastatic or residual RCC, regardless of the histologic type [24]. For this reason, adjuvant therapy is not currently recommended for children with translocation RCC and papillary RCC who have no residual tumor. Resection or irradiation of metastases can offer palliation for patients with bone or brain metastases [2].

There is no standard treatment for unresectable or metastatic RCC. High-dose interleukin-2 has had some success, but response is mainly observed in traditional clear-cell RCC, a very rare subtype in children [14]. In primary RCCs, response is found in 21% of patients with clear-cell versus 6% in patients with variant- or indeterminate-type RCC [51]. The recent advent of targeted therapies has significantly transformed the outcomes for patients with adult RCC. Several targeted therapies (e.g., sunitinib, sorafenib, bevacizumab, pazopanib, temsirolimus, and everolimus) have been approved for use in adults with RCC; however, these agents have not been tested in Paediatric patients with RCC. Inhibition of the VEGF pathway, by blocking the binding of VEGF to its receptor (i.e., bevacizumab) or by inhibiting the tyrosine kinase activity of the intracellular domain of the VEGF receptor with small molecules (i.e., sunitinib, sorafenib and pazopanib), has emerged as the primary therapeutic intervention for most patients with advanced RCC. In addition to targeting VEGF, the approved tyrosine kinase inhibitors target other pathways including FGFR, PDGFR, c-met, and AXL [52]. The mTOR is another molecular target for which small molecule inhibitors (i.e., temsirolimus and everolimus) have demonstrated a significant clinical activity in patients with advanced RCC. There is no absolute cross-resistance among the tyrosine kinase inhibitors, and this phenomenon appears to also be true between the VEGF pathway inhibitors and mTOR inhibitors. Currently, sequential single-agent therapy with targeted therapy has become the standard of care for metastatic RCC [53]. In Xp11 translocation RCC, targeted therapy achieved objective responses and prolonged progression-free survival similar to those reported for clear-cell RCC [54]. Furthermore, new immunotherapy strategies for RCC are emerging [32, 52]. Nivolumab, a programmed death 1 (PD-1) checkpoint inhibitor, showed longer overall survival and higher objective response rates than everolimus in patients with advanced clear-cell RCC who were previously treated with antiangiogenic therapy [55]. The COG is planning a prospective therapeutic trial in collaboration with adult cooperative groups for translocation RCC that affects primarily adolescents and young adults [56].

Renal medullary carcinoma is characterized by a high stage and lack of response to both chemotherapy and radiotherapy [33, 57]. Mortality approaches 100%, and death usually occurs within a few months of the diagnosis. Significant initial responses to cisplatin or carboplatin in combination with gemcitabine and paclitaxel have been rarely observed in renal medullary carcinoma [58].

3.8   Patient Outcomes and Prognosis

The 5-year survival rate for adults with RCC is approximately 75% [2], and the 1-year and 5-year survival rates for children with RCC are 87% and 70%, respectively [39]. Age and gender have no significant impact on survival. The major factor influencing the prognosis is the stage [38]. Patients with a localized stage (stage I and II) have the best prognosis; both the estimated 20-year event-free survival and overall survival rates for patients with stage I to II disease are 88.9% [38]. In addition, the reported 5-year survival estimates for children with stage I–IV RCC range from 93%–100%, 85%–91%, 71%–73%, and 8%–13%, respectively [39, 40]. The lung and liver are the most common sites of distant metastases and are usually fatal [38]. Survival is negatively impacted by increased tumor size and higher pathologic stage [39]. The importance of nodal status in children with RCC is controversial [39]. The systematic review of the literature found that 42 of 58 (72%) Paediatric patients with local lymph node involvement survived without evidence of disease at the last follow-up [40], whereas the National Cancer Database study found the 5-year survival to be decreased for children with positive nodes (55%) compared to children with negative nodes (83%) [39]. When compared to similar adult patients, the outcome of children with local lymph node involvement appears to be better, suggesting that Paediatric RCC, or the host, may present critical differences [40, 50]. Due to the rarity of Paediatric RCC, national and international collaborations are needed to conduct research that advances our knowledge about this disease, its biology, and treatment.

References

1. Eble JS, Sauter G, Epstein JI, Sesterhenn IA. Tumors of the kidney. In: World Health Organization classification of tumours. Pathology and genetics of tumours of the urinary system and male genital organs. Lyon: IARC Press; 2004. p. 9–87.
2. Doehn C, Grunwald V, Steiner T, Follmann M, Rexer H, Krege S. The diagnosis, treatment, and follow-up of renal cell carcinoma. Dtsch Arztebl Int. 2016;113(35–36):590–6.
3. Siegel DA, King J, Tai E, Buchanan N, Ajani UA, Li J. Cancer incidence rates and trends among children and adolescents in the United States, 2001–2009. Pediatrics. 2014;134(4):e945–55.
4. Akhavan A, Richards M, Shnorhavorian M, Goldin A, Gow K, Merguerian PA. Renal cell carcinoma in children, adolescents and young adults: a National Cancer Database study. J Urol. 2015;193(4):1336–41.
5. Wilms tumor and other childhood kidney tumors treatment (PDQ(R)): Health professional version. In: PDQ cancer information summaries. Bethesda, MD: National Cancer Institute; 2002.
6. Bernstein LLM, Smith MA, Olshan AF. Cancer incidence and survival among children and adolescents: United States SEER Program 1975–1995. Bethesda, MD: National Cancer Institute, SEER Program; 1999.
7. Geller JI, Ehrlich PF, Cost NG, et al. Characterization of adolescent and pediatric renal cell carcinoma: a report from the Children's Oncology Group study AREN03B2. Cancer. 2015;121(14):2457–64.
8. Chow WH, Dong LM, Devesa SS. Epidemiology and risk factors for kidney cancer. Nat Rev Urol. 2010;7(5):245–57.
9. Hunt JD, van der Hel OL, McMillan GP, Boffetta P, Brennan P. Renal cell carcinoma in relation to cigarette smoking: meta-analysis of 24 studies. Int J Cancer. 2005;114(1):101–8.

10. Chow WH, Gridley G, Fraumeni JF Jr, Jarvholm B. Obesity, hypertension, and the risk of kidney cancer in men. N Engl J Med. 2000;343(18):1305–11.
11. Silberstein J, Grabowski J, Saltzstein SL, Kane CJ. Renal cell carcinoma in the pediatric population: results from the California Cancer Registry. Pediatr Blood Cancer. 2009;52(2):237–41.
12. Selle B, Furtwangler R, Graf N, Kaatsch P, Bruder E, Leuschner I. Population-based study of renal cell carcinoma in children in Germany, 1980-2005: more frequently localized tumors and underlying disorders compared with adult counterparts. Cancer. 2006;107(12):2906–14.
13. Cohen D, Zhou M. Molecular genetics of familial renal cell carcinoma syndromes. Clin Lab Med. 2005;25(2):259–77.
14. Brok J, Treger TD, Gooskens SL, van den Heuvel-Eibrink MM, Pritchard-Jones K. Biology and treatment of renal tumours in childhood. Eur J Cancer. 2016;68:179–95.
15. Linehan WM, Srinivasan R, Schmidt LS. The genetic basis of kidney cancer: a metabolic disease. Nat Rev Urol. 2010;7(5):277–85.
16. Bjornsson J, Short MP, Kwiatkowski DJ, Henske EP. Tuberous sclerosis-associated renal cell carcinoma. Clinical, pathological, and genetic features. Am J Pathol. 1996;149(4):1201–8.
17. Nickerson ML, Warren MB, Toro JR, et al. Mutations in a novel gene lead to kidney tumors, lung wall defects, and benign tumors of the hair follicle in patients with the Birt–Hogg–Dube syndrome. Cancer Cell. 2002;2(2):157–64.
18. Tomlinson IP, Alam NA, Rowan AJ, et al. Germline mutations in FH predispose to dominantly inherited uterine fibroids, skin leiomyomata and papillary renal cell cancer. Nat Genet. 2002;30(4):406–10.
19. Menko FH, Maher ER, Schmidt LS, et al. Hereditary leiomyomatosis and renal cell cancer (HLRCC): renal cancer risk, surveillance and treatment. Familial Cancer. 2014;13(4):637–44.
20. Schmidt L, Duh FM, Chen F, et al. Germline and somatic mutations in the tyrosine kinase domain of the MET proto-oncogene in papillary renal carcinomas. Nat Genet. 1997;16(1):68–73.
21. Lubensky IA, Schmidt L, Zhuang Z, et al. Hereditary and sporadic papillary renal carcinomas with c-met mutations share a distinct morphological phenotype. Am J Pathol. 1999;155(2):517–26.
22. Watanabe IC, Billis A, Guimaraes MS, et al. Renal medullary carcinoma: report of seven cases from Brazil. Mod Pathol. 2007;20(9):914–20.
23. Moch H, Cubilla AL, Humphrey PA, Reuter VE, Ulbright TM. The 2016 WHO classification of tumours of the urinary system and male genital organs-part a: renal, penile, and testicular tumours. Eur Urol. 2016;70(1):93–105.
24. Perlman EJ. Pediatric renal cell carcinoma. Surg Pathol Clin. 2010;3(3):641–51.
25. Lopez-Beltran A, Scarpelli M, Montironi R, Kirkali Z. 2004 WHO classification of the renal tumors of the adults. Eur Urol. 2006;49(5):798–805.
26. Bruder E, Passera O, Harms D, et al. Morphologic and molecular characterization of renal cell carcinoma in children and young adults. Am J Surg Pathol. 2004;28(9):1117–32.
27. Argani P, Ladanyi M. Translocation carcinomas of the kidney. Clin Lab Med. 2005;25(2):363–78.
28. Geller JI, Argani P, Adeniran A, et al. Translocation renal cell carcinoma: lack of negative impact due to lymph node spread. Cancer. 2008;112(7):1607–16.
29. Argani P, Ladanyi M. The evolving story of renal translocation carcinomas. Am J Clin Pathol. 2006;126(3):332–4.
30. Hirobe M, Masumori N, Tanaka T, et al. Clinicopathological characteristics of Xp11.2 translocation renal cell carcinoma in adolescents and adults: Diagnosis using immunostaining of transcription factor E3 and fluorescence in situ hybridization analysis. Int J Urol. 2016;23(2):140–5.
31. Delahunt B, Eble JN, McCredie MR, Bethwaite PB, Stewart JH, Bilous AM. Morphologic typing of papillary renal cell carcinoma: comparison of growth kinetics and patient survival in 66 cases. Hum Pathol. 2001;32(6):590–5.
32. Dutcher JP. Recent developments in the treatment of renal cell carcinoma. Ther Adv Urol. 2013;5(6):338–53.
33. Swartz MA, Karth J, Schneider DT, Rodriguez R, Beckwith JB, Perlman EJ. Renal medullary carcinoma: clinical, pathologic, immunohistochemical, and genetic analysis with pathogenetic implications. Urology. 2002;60(6):1083–9.

34. Wallace B, Organ M, Bagnell S, Rendon R, Merrimen J. Renal cell carcinoma after neuroblastoma: a case study and review of the literature. Can Urol Assoc J. 2015;9(5–6):E316–8.
35. Medeiros LJ, Palmedo G, Krigman HR, Kovacs G, Beckwith JB. Oncocytoid renal cell carcinoma after neuroblastoma: a report of four cases of a distinct clinicopathologic entity. Am J Surg Pathol. 1999;23(7):772–80.
36. Hedgepeth RC, Zhou M, Ross J. Rapid development of metastatic Xp11 translocation renal cell carcinoma in a girl treated for neuroblastoma. J Pediatr Hematol Oncol. 2009;31(8):602–4.
37. Delahunt B, Cheville JC, Martignoni G, et al. The International Society of Urological Pathology (ISUP) grading system for renal cell carcinoma and other prognostic parameters. Am J Surg Pathol. 2013;37(10):1490–504.
38. Indolfi P, Terenziani M, Casale F, et al. Renal cell carcinoma in children: a clinicopathologic study. J Clin Oncol. 2003;21(3):530–5.
39. Rialon KL, Gulack BC, Englum BR, Routh JC, Rice HE. Factors impacting survival in children with renal cell carcinoma. J Pediatr Surg. 2015;50(6):1014–8.
40. Geller JI, Dome JS. Local lymph node involvement does not predict poor outcome in pediatric renal cell carcinoma. Cancer. 2004;101(7):1575–83.
41. Spreafico F, Collini P, Terenziani M, Marchiano A, Piva L. Renal cell carcinoma in children and adolescents. Expert Rev Anticancer Ther. 2010;10(12):1967–78.
42. Stenzl A, de Kernion JB. Pathology, biology, and clinical staging of renal cell carcinoma. Semin Oncol. 1989;16(1 Suppl 1):3–11.
43. Carcao MD, Taylor GP, Greenberg ML, et al. Renal-cell carcinoma in children: a different disorder from its adult counterpart? Med Pediatr Oncol. 1998;31(3):153–8.
44. Laski ME, Vugrin D. Paraneoplastic syndromes in hypernephroma. Semin Nephrol. 1987;7(2):123–30.
45. Lee EY. CT imaging of mass-like renal lesions in children. Pediatr Radiol. 2007;37(9):896–907.
46. Malkan AD, Loh A, Bahrami A, et al. An approach to renal masses in pediatrics. Pediatrics. 2015;135(1):142–58.
47. Gow KW, Barnhart DC, Hamilton TE, et al. Primary nephrectomy and intraoperative tumor spill: report from the Children's Oncology Group (COG) renal tumors committee. J Pediatr Surg. 2013;48(1):34–8.
48. Skoldenberg EG, Jakobson A, Elvin A, Sandstedt B, Lackgren G, Christofferson RH. Pretreatment, ultrasound-guided cutting needle biopsies in childhood renal tumors. Med Pediatr Oncol. 1999;32(4):283–8.
49. Volpe A, Jewett MA. Current role, techniques and outcomes of percutaneous biopsy of renal tumors. Expert Rev Anticancer Ther. 2009;9(6):773–83.
50. Indolfi P, Bisogno G, Cecchetto G, et al. Local lymph node involvement in pediatric renal cell carcinoma: a report from the Italian TREP project. Pediatr Blood Cancer. 2008;51(4):475–8.
51. Upton MP, Parker RA, Youmans A, McDermott DF, Atkins MB. Histologic predictors of renal cell carcinoma response to interleukin-2-based therapy. J Immunother. 2005;28(5):488–95.
52. Choueiri TK, Motzer RJ. Systemic therapy for metastatic renal-cell carcinoma. N Engl J Med. 2017;376(4):354–66.
53. Battelli C, Cho DC. mTOR inhibitors in renal cell carcinoma. Therapy. 2011;8(4):359–67.
54. Malouf GG, Camparo P, Oudard S, et al. Targeted agents in metastatic Xp11 translocation/TFE3 gene fusion renal cell carcinoma (RCC): a report from the Juvenile RCC Network. Ann Oncol. 2010;21(9):1834–8.
55. Motzer RJ, Escudier B, McDermott DF, et al. Nivolumab versus everolimus in advanced renal-cell carcinoma. N Engl J Med. 2015;373(19):1803–13.
56. Dome JS, Fernandez CV, Mullen EA, et al. Children's Oncology Group's 2013 blueprint for research: renal tumors. Pediatr Blood Cancer. 2013;60(6):994–1000.
57. Avery RA, Harris JE, Davis CJ Jr, Borgaonkar DS, Byrd JC, Weiss RB. Renal medullary carcinoma: clinical and therapeutic aspects of a newly described tumor. Cancer. 1996;78(1):128–32.
58. Strouse JJ, Spevak M, Mack AK, Arceci RJ, Small D, Loeb DM. Significant responses to platinum-based chemotherapy in renal medullary carcinoma. Pediatr Blood Cancer. 2005;44(4):407–11.

Chromophobe Renal Cell Carcinoma

4

Aaron R. Lim and W. Kimryn Rathmell

4.1 Defining Chromophobe Renal Cell Carcinoma

Chromophobe renal cell carcinoma (ChRCC) makes up approximately 5% of all cases of renal cell carcinoma (RCC) [1]. First described in 1985, this rare subtype of RCC was originally thought to arise from the intercalated cells of the collecting ducts. This disease is challenging to diagnose, and on biopsy, this malignancy can share histologic similarities with benign oncocytomas using conventional evaluation or even be misclassified as the more common clear-cell RCC [2–4]. Therefore, careful histologic attention is needed to appropriately capture these cases. Histologically, two variants of ChRCC are recognized: classic ChRCC and an eosinophilic variant [5]. The classic type is more common and is characterized by large cells with pale "chromophobe" cytoplasm and a perinuclear halo or clearing. On the other hand, the tumor cells in the eosinophilic variant display a dense eosinophilic cytoplasm and perinuclear halos (Fig. 4.1).

Karyotyping studies have recognized for some time that there is a characteristic pattern of chromosome loss that is recurrent in this disease [6, 7]. The high-frequency loss of one copy of chromosomes 1, 2, 6, 10, 13, and 17 remains a conundrum that will be discussed in detail below. Recent genetic analysis of ChRCC by The Cancer Genome Atlas (TCGA) confirmed this unique genomic landscape that distinguishes this rare subtype from clear-cell renal cell carcinoma (ccRCC) and papillary renal cell carcinoma (pRCC). In addition to the large-scale loss of multiple chromosomes, this disease is also characterized by high frequency of mutations in *TP53* and *PTEN* [8]. Although most cases of ChRCC occur sporadically, a subset of patients with tuberous sclerosis complex and Birt-Hogg-Dubé syndrome develop a renal neoplasm consistent with a chromophobe histology [9, 10].

A. R. Lim · W. K. Rathmell (✉)
Vanderbilt-Ingram Cancer Center, Nashville, TN, USA
e-mail: Kimryn.rathmell@vanderbilt.edu

© Springer Nature Switzerland AG 2019

43

G. G. Malouf, N. M. Tannir (eds.), *Rare Kidney Tumors*,
https://doi.org/10.1007/978-3-319-96989-3_4

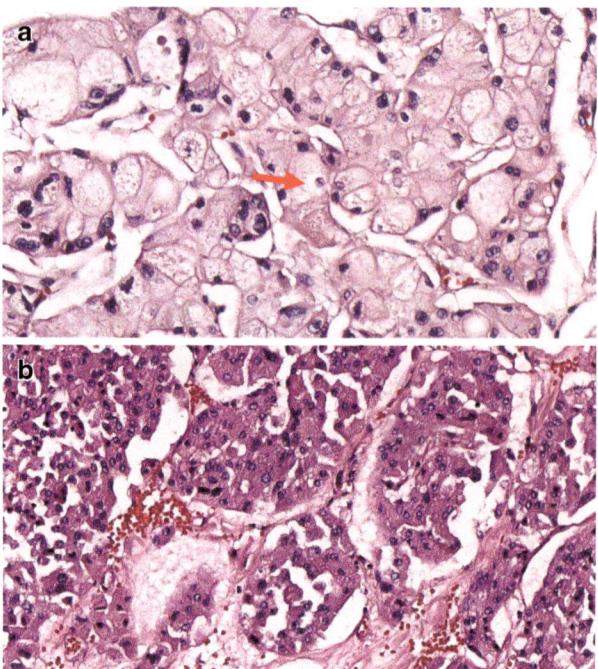

Fig. 4.1 Pathology of classic and eosinophilic ChRCC. (**a**) A representative H&E stain of a classic ChRCC highlighting cells with pale cytoplasm and a perinuclear halo (red arrow). (**b**) A representative H&E stain of an eosinophilic variant of ChRCC showing crowded cells with eosinophilic cytoplasm (images obtained from http://cancer.digitalslidearchive.net, TCGA-KL-8324-01Z-00-DX1, TCGA-KN-8436-01Z-00-DX1)

Clinical staging of ChRCC is derived from other forms of RCC. However, Fuhrman grading, which is used for grading ccRCC, does not provide prognostic value for ChRCC [11, 12]. Although other grading systems for ChRCC have been developed, these other systems have not been rigorously tested [13]. Thus, the International Society of Urologic Pathology recommends that ChRCC should be not be graded [14].

4.2 Genomic Landscape of Chromophobe Renal Cell Carcinoma

An important genetic feature of ChRCC, introduced above, is the loss of numerous chromosomes (Fig. 4.2). Copy number analysis of 66 ChRCC samples in the TCGA showed frequent loss of chromosomes 1, 2, 6, 10, 13, and 17 [8]. Less frequently, but still at significantly higher frequency than observed in other tumors, chromosomes 3, 5, 8, 9, 11, 18, and 21 show evidence of loss [8]. The reason behind the extensive loss of genomic material remains unknown.

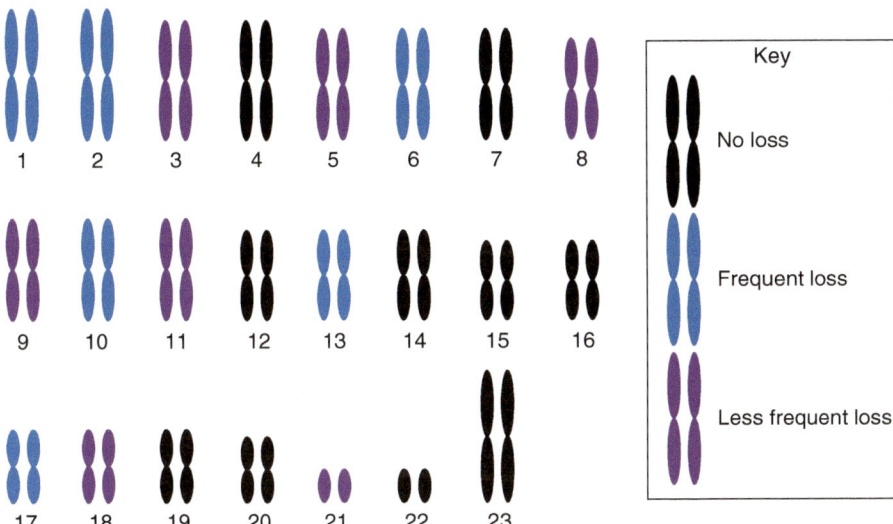

Fig. 4.2 Hypodiploidy in ChRCC. Chromosomes 1, 2, 6, 10, 13, and 17 are frequently lost in ChRCC (blue chromosomes). Chromosomes 3, 5, 8, 9, 11, 18, and 21 are less frequently lost in ChRCC (purple chromosomes), though still at an elevated rate compared to other tumors

Using whole exome sequencing, the TCGA demonstrated that *TP53* is the most commonly mutated gene in ChRCC. It is notable that this common tumor suppressor is rarely mutated in ccRCC and pRCC [8]. Along with frequent loss of chromosome 17, frequent *TP53* mutation suggests that deficiency of p53 may be one feature driving ChRCC tumorigenesis. The second most commonly mutated gene in ChRCC identified by the TCGA is *PTEN* [8]. In combination with frequent loss of chromosome 10, complete absence of PTEN points to constitutive activation of the PI3K/AKT/mTOR signaling pathway in ChRCC, which may explain the efficacy of mTOR inhibitors in ChRCC [8].

Interestingly, a subset of tumors in the TCGA showed increased expression of telomerase, which is encoded by the *TERT* gene. Unexpectedly, whole genome sequencing revealed that the tumors with the highest telomerase expression had genomic breakpoints within the *TERT* promoter leading to structural rearrangement [8]. This finding has spawned a new search for structural variants due to mutations outside the TERT open reading frame that can alter TERT protein levels.

In addition to these distinctions, expression-based profiling has demonstrated that these tumors share transcriptional features most consistent with a distal tubule origin, when compared with microdissected kidney tubule segments [15, 16]. This is in contrast to both clear-cell and papillary-type RCC, which map more closely to the proximal tubule segments. Taken together, these genomic features unique to ChRCC support the argument that ChRCC is a completely different cancer, derived from a separate geographic region of the nephron and with a distinct mutational profile, that distinguishes this malignancy from the other RCC subtypes [17].

4.3   Hereditary Forms of Chromophobe Renal Cell Carcinoma

Several genetic conditions have been associated with the development of ChRCC, including Birt-Hogg-Dubé (BHD) syndrome and tuberous sclerosis complex (TSC). Named after three physicians who described it in a Canadian family in 1977, BHD syndrome is an autosomal dominant condition characterized by fibrofolliculomas, pulmonary cysts, spontaneous pneumothorax, and kidney neoplasms [18, 19]. Approximately 12–34% of BHD patients will develop a renal neoplasm, 40% of which are ChRCC [10, 20, 21]. Other renal tumors found in this syndrome include oncocytomas, hybrid oncocytic/chromophobe tumors, and ccRCC [22]. Genetically, patients with BHD syndrome harbor germline mutations in the tumor suppressor gene *FLCN*, which is rarely mutated in sporadic cases of ChRCC [23–25]. The majority of these mutations result in truncation of the folliculin protein [20, 26]. Numerous functions of folliculin have been proposed, including regulating AKT/mTOR and TGFβ signaling, sequestering transcription factor E3 in the cytoplasm, and facilitating cell-cell adhesion [27–31]. However, further studies are needed to elucidate the connection between the functions of this tumor suppressor and the manifestations of BHD syndrome.

TSC is an autosomal dominant condition that results from mutations in either *TSC1* or *TSC2,* causing severe neurologic dysfunction and tumors in the brain, kidney, skin, heart, and lung [32, 33]. Inactivating either of these tumor suppressor genes leads to increased activation of mTOR signaling and cellular proliferation [34]. Renal disease in TSC, which is the second leading cause of death in these patients, includes renal angiomyolipomas, renal cysts, and RCC [35]. Although patients with TSC have a similar incidence of RCC as the general population (2–3%), they tend to develop these tumors at a median age of 28 years, which is 25 years younger than the general population [35, 36]. A recent study of 46 renal tumors from TSC patients showed that 33% contained a hybrid oncocytic/chromophobe phenotype, though it is important to note that TSC-associated RCCs encompass other histologic subtypes including ccRCC and pRCC [36–38].

4.4   Metabolism of Chromophobe Renal Cell Carcinoma

It had previously been shown that mitochondrial DNA was altered in both oncocytomas and the eosinophilic variant of ChRCC, both of which have been known to contain an abundance of mitochondria [39, 40]. The TCGA extended their analysis of ChRCC to include mitochondrial DNA and found that 18% of their ChRCC tumors had mutations leading to inactivation of the electron transport chain (ETC) complex I [8]. *MT-ND5*, which encodes an essential component of ETC complex I called NADH dehydrogenase 5, was the most frequently altered mitochondrial gene and correlated strongly with the eosinophilic ChRCC variant [8, 41]. However, mutations in ETC complex I did not correlate with loss of oxidative phosphorylation [8]. It remains to be determined whether inactivation of ETC complex I triggers increased mitochondrial abundance as a compensatory mechanism or if it leads to an alternative metabolic route to support ChRCC.

4.5 Clinical Aspects and Management of Chromophobe Renal Cell Carcinoma

ChRCC has a more favorable prognosis than ccRCC and pRCC, with 5-year survival rates ranging from 78% to 100% [42]. This beneficial survival stems largely from the overall better prognosis for localized disease, which generally shows low risk for metastatic spread. Although most cases of ChRCC remain localized, metastatic cases of ChRCC have been known to occur [43, 44]. However, only 1.3% of patients with ChRCC present with metastatic disease, and they usually have a better prognosis compared to patients with other metastatic RCC subtypes [45, 46]. Factors that predict worse prognosis include sarcomatoid dedifferentiation, microscopic necrosis, and advanced stage [42].

Due to the rarity of ChRCC, studies on how to manage patients with ChRCC are scarce. ChRCC patients are usually managed similarly to ccRCC patients, with localized disease being treated with surgical resection. Surgical guidelines for the management of this cancer are applied from those developed for ccRCC. Advanced ChRCC remains difficult to treat, and it is strongly recommended to enroll these patients into chromophobe-specific clinical trials [47]. Most studies that investigate treatment for RCC exclude non-ccRCC patients, and those that include non-ccRCC subtypes are usually made up of mostly pRCC patients with a small number of ChRCC patients.

Historical therapies such as interferon and IL-2 have not been shown to be efficacious in advanced ChRCC. For example, in a study of 64 patients with metastatic non-ccRCC, only one of the 12 patients with metastatic ChRCC responded to interferon alpha 2a, IL-2, or combination of interferon alpha 2a and IL-2 therapy [46]. Chemotherapy is of limited use in the renal cell carcinomas, as discussed elsewhere in this text. A phase II trial showed that only one out of seven patients with ChRCC had a complete response to capecitabine monotherapy [48]. Thus, systemic chemotherapy is not currently recommended for advanced ChRCC, although the new data demonstrating the strong association with TP53 mutations is rekindling interest in the possibility for chemotherapy to be reinvestigated in this disease.

On the other hand, patients with advanced ChRCC have been shown to respond to the targeted therapies that are widely used in ccRCC, such as vascular endothelial growth factor receptor (VEGFR) inhibitors and mTOR inhibitors. One study showed that 25% of metastatic ChRCC patients in five US and French institutions had clinical response to VEGFR inhibitors sunitinib and sorafenib compared to only 5% of metastatic pRCC patients [49]. Similar results were demonstrated in a recent phase II trial which showed that metastatic ChRCC patients treated with sunitinib had a 40% response rate and a median progression-free survival of 12.7 months [50].

Since *PTEN* mutations and loss of chromosome 10 have been found in ChRCC, mTOR inhibitors have a strong biological rationale and have been investigated as potential therapies for ChRCC patients. A subtype group analysis from the phase III global advanced renal cell carcinoma (ARCC) trial demonstrated that temsirolimus had superior efficacy compared to interferon in non-ccRCC subtypes [51]. In addition, ChRCC patients in a recent phase II Korean study had a median progression-free survival of 13.1 months on everolimus, whereas pRCC patients had a median progression-free survival of only 3.4 months [52]. In the ESPN trial comparing everolimus and sunitinib, neither drug showed superiority as a first-line therapy for metastatic non-ccRCC [53]. However, the ASPEN trial, which included more patients than the ESPN trial, concluded that metastatic ChRCC patients treated with everolimus had longer median progression-free survival compared to those treated with sunitinib, which was the opposite result they saw for pRCC patients [54]. Taken together, these trials show that both VEGFR and mTOR inhibitors may provide therapeutic benefit to patients with advanced ChRCC, though future studies should investigate molecular biomarkers that can predict response to targeted therapies.

Other therapies such as radiation therapy and immune checkpoint blockade have not been extensively studied in ChRCC. There is no clear role for using radiation to treat ChRCC except as a means for palliative care. Although immune checkpoint inhibitors such as Nivolumab, a monoclonal antibody targeting PD-1, have demonstrated efficacy in ccRCC, their efficacy in ChRCC remains unknown. Choueiri et al. recently characterized PD-L1 expression in non-ccRCC tumors and found that patients with PD-L1+ tumors have worse prognoses [55]. In addition, there is currently a clinical trial investigating Nivolumab's efficacy and safety in advanced non-ccRCC patients (ClinicalTrials.gov Identifier: NCT02596035). Thus, immune checkpoint blockade represents an interesting area of future study for ChRCC.

Conclusion

ChRCC is a rare subtype of RCC that is usually indolent compared to the other RCC subtypes. With the TCGA's recent comprehensive genetic analysis of ChRCC, we have learned that ChRCC has distinct genomic features, including an unprecedented loss of numerous chromosomes, mutations in *TP53* and *PTEN*, rearrangements in the *TERT* promoter, and mutations in mitochondrial DNA. BHD syndrome and TSC are two examples of genetic syndromes that predispose individuals to developing ChRCC, though most ChRCC cases are sporadic. These unique genomic characteristics underscore the importance of distinguishing ChRCC from the other RCC subtypes. Even though there is strong evidence to consider ChRCC as a separate disease from ccRCC, we currently do not have separate treatment guidelines for ChRCC. Although recent clinical trials have shown that advanced ChRCC patients may respond to targeted therapy such as VEGFR and mTOR inhibitors, current studies that have non-ccRCC patients are dominated by pRCC patients and simply do not enroll enough ChRCC patients due to its rarity. Thus, it is prudent to further our understanding of its molecular biology and establish clinical trials that include more ChRCC patients in order to develop better therapies for this distinct disease entity.

References

1. Lopez-Beltran A, Carrasco JC, Cheng L, Scarpelli M, Kirkali Z, Montironi R. 2009 Update on the classification of renal epithelial tumors in adults. Int J Urol. 2009;16(5):432–43. https://doi.org/10.1111/j.1442-2042.2009.02302.x.
2. Thoenes W, Storkel S, Rumpelt HJ. Human chromophobe cell renal carcinoma. Virchows Arch B Cell Pathol Incl Mol Pathol. 1985;48(3):207–17.
3. Störkel S, Steart PV, Drenckhahn D, Thoenes W. The human chromophobe cell renal carcinoma: Its probable relation to intercalated cells of the collecting duct. Virchows Arch B Cell Pathol Incl Mol Pathol. 1988;56(1):237–45. https://doi.org/10.1007/BF02890022.
4. Delongchamps NB, Galmiche L, Eiss D, et al. Hybrid tumour "oncocytoma-chromophobe renal cell carcinoma" of the kidney: A report of seven sporadic cases. BJU Int. 2009;103(10):1381–4. https://doi.org/10.1111/j.1464-410X.2008.08263.x.
5. Podduturi V, Yourshaw CJ, Zhang H. Eosinophilic variant of chromophobe renal cell carcinoma. Proc (Bayl Univ Med Cent). 2015;28(1):57–8.
6. Speicher MR, Schoell B, du Manoir S, et al. Specific loss of chromosomes 1, 2, 6, 10, 13, 17, and 21 in chromophobe renal cell carcinomas revealed by comparative genomic hybridization. Am J Pathol. 1994;145(2):356–64.
7. Iqbal MA, Akhtar M, Ali MA. Cytogenetic findings in renal cell carcinoma. Hum Pathol. 1996;27(9):949–54.
8. Davis CF, Ricketts CJ, Wang M, et al. The somatic genomic landscape of chromophobe renal cell carcinoma. Cancer Cell. 2014;26(3):319–30. https://doi.org/10.1016/j.ccr.2014.07.014.
9. Guo J, Tretiakova MS, Troxell ML, et al. Tuberous sclerosis-associated renal cell carcinoma: a clinicopathologic study of 57 separate carcinomas in 18 patients. Am J Surg Pathol. 2014;38(11):1457–67. https://doi.org/10.1097/PAS.0000000000000248.
10. Pavlovich CP, Walther MM, Eyler RA, et al. Renal tumors in the Birt-Hogg-Dubé syndrome. Am J Surg Pathol. 2002;26(12):1542–52. https://doi.org/10.1097/00000478-200212000-00002.
11. Delahunt B, Sika-Paotonu D, Bethwaite PB, et al. Fuhrman grading is not appropriate for chromophobe renal cell carcinoma. Am J Surg Pathol. 2007;31(6):957–60. https://doi.org/10.1097/01.pas.0000249446.28713.53.
12. Steffens S, Janssen M, Roos FC, et al. The Fuhrman grading system has no prognostic value in patients with nonsarcomatoid chromophobe renal cell carcinoma. Hum Pathol. 2014;45(12):2411–6. https://doi.org/10.1016/j.humpath.2014.08.002.
13. Paner GP, Amin MB, Alvarado-Cabrero I, et al. A novel tumor grading scheme for chromophobe renal cell carcinoma: prognostic utility and comparison with Fuhrman nuclear grade. Am J Surg Pathol. 2010;34(9):1233–40. https://doi.org/10.1097/PAS.0b013e3181e96f2a.
14. Delahunt B, Cheville JC, Martignoni G, et al. The International Society of Urological Pathology (ISUP) grading system for renal cell carcinoma and other prognostic parameters. Am J Surg Pathol. 2013;37(10):1490–504. https://doi.org/10.1097/PAS.0b013e318299f0fb.
15. Prasad SR, Narra VR, Shah R, et al. Segmental disorders of the nephron: histopathological and imaging perspective. Br J Radiol. 2007;80(956):593–602. https://doi.org/10.1259/bjr/20129205.
16. Chen F, Zhang Y, Senbabaoglu Y, et al. Multilevel genomics-based taxonomy of renal cell carcinoma. Cell Rep. 2016;14(10):2476–89. https://doi.org/10.1016/j.celrep.2016.02.024.
17. Fahey CC, Rathmell WK. A tale of two cancers: Complete genetic analysis of chromophobe renal cell carcinoma contrasts with clear cell renal cell carcinoma. Mol Cell Oncol. 2015;2(2):e979686. https://doi.org/10.4161/23723556.2014.979686.
18. Birt AR, Hogg GR, Dubé WJ, et al. Hereditary multiple fibrofolliculomas with trichodiscomas and acrochordons. Arch Dermatol. 1977;113(12):1674. https://doi.org/10.1001/archderm.1977.01640120042005.
19. Schmidt LS, Warren MB, Nickerson ML, et al. Birt-Hogg-Dubé syndrome, a genodermatosis associated with spontaneous pneumothorax and kidney neoplasia, maps to chromosome 17p11.2. Am J Hum Genet. 2001;69(4):876–82. https://doi.org/10.1086/323744.

20. Schmidt LS, Linehan WM. Molecular genetics and clinical features of Birt–Hogg–Dubé syndrome. Nat Rev Urol. 2015;12(10):558–69. https://doi.org/10.1038/nrurol.2015.206.
21. Rathmell KW, Chen F, Creighton CJ. Genomics of chromophobe renal cell carcinoma: implications from a rare tumor for pan-cancer studies. Oncoscience. 2015;2(2):81–90. https://doi.org/10.18632/oncoscience.130.
22. Lara PN, Jonasch E, editors. Kidney cancer. 2nd ed. New York: Springer International Publishing; 2015. https://doi.org/10.1007/978-3-319-17903-2.
23. Nickerson ML, Warren MB, Toro JR, et al. Mutations in a novel gene lead to kidney tumors, lung wall defects, and benign tumors of the hair follicle in patients with the Birt-Hogg-Dubé syndrome. Cancer Cell. 2002;2(2):157–64. https://doi.org/10.1016/S1535-6108(02)00104-6.
24. Nagy A, Zoubakov D, Stupar Z, Kovacs G. Lack of mutation of the folliculin gene in sporadic chromophobe renal cell carcinoma and renal oncocytoma. Int J Cancer. 2004;109(3):472–5. https://doi.org/10.1002/ijc.11694.
25. Khoo SK, Kahnoski K, Sugimura J, et al. Inactivation of BHD in sporadic renal tumors. Cancer Res. 2003;63(15):4583–7.
26. Lim DHK, Rehal PK, Nahorski MS, et al. A new locus-specific database (LSDB) for mutations in the folliculin (FLCN) gene. Hum Mutat. 2010;31(1):E1043–51. https://doi.org/10.1002/humu.21130.
27. Tsun Z-Y, Bar-Peled L, Chantranupong L, et al. The folliculin tumor suppressor is a GAP for the RagC/D GTPases that signal amino acid levels to mTORC1. Mol Cell. 2013;52(4):495–505. https://doi.org/10.1016/j.molcel.2013.09.016.
28. Hong SB, Oh H, Valera VA, et al. Tumor suppressor FLCN inhibits tumorigenesis of a FLCN-null renal cancer cell line and regulates expression of key molecules in TGF-β signaling. Mol Cancer. 2010;9(1):160. https://doi.org/10.1186/1476-4598-9-160.
29. Hong SB, Oh H, Valera VA, Baba M, Schmidt LS, Linehan WM. Inactivation of the FLCN tumor suppressor gene induces TFE3 transcriptional activity by increasing its nuclear localization. PLoS One. 2010;5(12):e15793. https://doi.org/10.1371/journal.pone.0015793.
30. Medvetz DA, Khabibullin D, Hariharan V, et al. Folliculin, the product of the Birt-Hogg-Dube tumor suppressor gene, interacts with the adherens junction protein p0071 to regulate cell-cell adhesion. PLoS One. 2012;7(11):e47842. https://doi.org/10.1371/journal.pone.0047842.
31. Nahorski MS, Seabra L, Straatman-Iwanowska A, et al. Folliculin interacts with p0071 (plakophilin-4) and deficiency is associated with disordered Rhoa signalling, epithelial polarization and cytokinesis. Hum Mol Genet. 2012;21(24):5268–79. https://doi.org/10.1093/hmg/dds378.
32. Northrup H, Krueger DA. Tuberous sclerosis complex diagnostic criteria update: Recommendations of the 2012 international tuberous sclerosis complex consensus conference. Pediatr Neurol. 2013;49(4):243–54. https://doi.org/10.1016/j.pediatrneurol.2013.08.001.
33. Curatolo P, Bombardieri R, Jozwiak S. Tuberous sclerosis. Lancet. 2008;372(9639):657–68. https://doi.org/10.1016/S0140-6736(08)61279-9.
34. Tee AR, Fingar DC, Manning BD, Kwiatkowski DJ, Cantley LC, Blenis J. Tuberous sclerosis complex-1 and -2 gene products function together to inhibit mammalian target of rapamycin (mTOR)-mediated downstream signaling. Proc Natl Acad Sci U S A. 2002;99(21):13571–6. https://doi.org/10.1073/pnas.202476899.
35. Crino PB, Nathanson KL, Henske EP. The tuberous sclerosis complex. N Engl J Med. 2006;355:1345–56. https://doi.org/10.1056/NEJMra055323.
36. Washecka R, Hanna M. Malignant renal tumors in tuberous sclerosis. Urology. 1991;37(4):340–3. https://doi.org/10.1016/0090-4295(91)80261-5.
37. Yang P, Cornejo K, Sadow P, Cheng L, Wang M, Wu C. Renal cell carcinoma in tuberous sclerosis complex. Am J Surg Pathol. 2014;38(7):895–909. https://doi.org/10.1097/PAS.0000000000000237.
38. Bjornsson J, Short MP, Kwiatkowski DJ, Henske EP. Tuberous sclerosis-associated renal cell carcinoma. Clinical, pathological, and genetic features. Am J Pathol. 1996;149(4):1201–8.
39. Welter C, Kovacs G, Seitz G, Blin N. Alteration of mitochondrial DNA in human oncocytomas. Genes Chromosomes Cancer. 1989;1(1):79–82.

40. Kovacs A, Storkel S, Thoenes W, Kovacs G. Mitochondrial and chromosomal DNA alterations in human chromophobe renal cell carcinomas. J Pathol. 1992;167(3):273–7. https://doi.org/10.1002/path.1711670303.
41. Chomyn A. Mitochondrial genetic control of assembly and function of complex I in mammalian cells. J Bioenerg Biomembr. 2001;33(3):251–7.
42. Amin MB, Paner GP, Alvarado-Cabrero I, et al. Chromophobe renal cell carcinoma: histomorphologic characteristics and evaluation of conventional pathologic prognostic parameters in 145 cases. Am J Surg Pathol. 2008;32(12):1822–34. https://doi.org/10.1097/PAS.0b013e3181831e68.
43. Thoenes W, Störkel S, Rumpelt HJ, Moll R, Baum HP, Werner S. Chromophobe cell renal carcinoma and its variants--a report on 32 cases. J Pathol. 1988;155(4):277–87. https://doi.org/10.1002/path.1711550402.
44. Crotty TB, Farrow GM, Lieber MM. Chromophobe cell renal carcinoma: Clinicopathological features of 50 cases. J Urol. 1995;154(3):964–7. https://doi.org/10.1016/S0022-5347(01)66944-1.
45. Volpe A, Novara G, Antonelli A, et al. Chromophobe renal cell carcinoma (RCC): Oncological outcomes and prognostic factors in a large multicentre series. BJU Int. 2012;110(1):76–83. https://doi.org/10.1111/j.1464-410X.2011.10690.x.
46. Motzer RJ, Bacik J, Mariani T, Russo P, Mazumdar M, Reuter V. Treatment outcome and survival associated with metastatic renal cell carcinoma of non-clear-cell histology. J Clin Oncol. 2002;20(9):2376–81. https://doi.org/10.1200/JCO.2002.11.123.
47. Escudier B, Porta C, Schmidinger M, et al. Renal cell carcinoma: ESMO Clinical Practice Guidelines for diagnosis, treatment and follow-up. Ann Oncol. 2016;27(suppl 5):v58–68. https://doi.org/10.1093/annonc/mdw328.
48. Tsimafeyeu I, Demidov L, Kharkevich G, et al. Phase II, multicenter, uncontrolled trial of single-agent capecitabine in patients with non-clear cell metastatic renal cell carcinoma. Am J Clin Oncol. 2012;35(3):251–4. https://doi.org/10.1097/COC.0b013e31820dbc17.
49. Choueiri TK, Plantade A, Elson P, et al. Efficacy of sunitinib and sorafenib in metastatic papillary and chromophobe renal cell carcinoma. J Clin Oncol. 2008;26(1):127–31. https://doi.org/10.1200/JCO.2007.13.3223.
50. Tannir NM, Plimack E, Ng C, et al. A phase 2 trial of sunitinib in patients with advanced non-clear cell renal cell carcinoma. Eur Urol. 2012;62(6):1013–9. https://doi.org/10.1016/j.eururo.2012.06.043.
51. Dutcher JP, De Souza P, McDermott D, et al. Effect of temsirolimus versus interferon-alpha on outcome of patients with advanced renal cell carcinoma of different tumor histologies. Med Oncol. 2009;26(2):202–9. https://doi.org/10.1007/s12032-009-9177-0.
52. Koh Y, Lim HY, Ahn JH, et al. Phase II trial of everolimus for the treatment of nonclear-cell renal cell carcinoma. Ann Oncol. 2013;24(4):1026–31. https://doi.org/10.1093/annonc/mds582.
53. Tannir NM, Jonasch E, Albiges L, et al. Everolimus versus sunitinib prospective evaluation in metastatic non-clear cell renal cell carcinoma (ESPN): A randomized multicenter phase 2 trial. Eur Urol. 2016;69(5):866–74. https://doi.org/10.1016/j.eururo.2015.10.049.
54. Armstrong AJ, Halabi S, Eisen T, et al. Everolimus versus sunitinib for patients with metastatic non-clear cell renal cell carcinoma (ASPEN): A multicentre, open-label, randomised phase 2 trial. Lancet Oncol. 2016;17(3):378–88. https://doi.org/10.1016/S1470-2045(15)00515-X.
55. Choueiri TK, Fay AP, Gray KP, et al. PD-L1 expression in nonclear-cell renal cell carcinoma. Ann Oncol. 2014;25(11):2178–84. https://doi.org/10.1093/annonc/mdu445.

Papillary Renal Cell Carcinoma

5

Ramaprasad Srinivasan and Kai Hammerich

5.1 Introduction

Papillary renal cell carcinoma (pRCC) is the second most common subtype of kidney cancer after clear cell renal cell carcinoma (ccRCC) and accounts for approximately 15–20% of renal malignancies [1, 2]. The term papillary RCC is a histologic designation, and the diagnosis is based on the presence of papillary or tubulopapillary structures on histopathologic evaluation. Historically, two histologic subtypes of papillary RCC, type 1 and type 2, have been recognized [3]; however, there is considerable histologic and molecular heterogeneity underlying this entity that transcends this simple histologic classification [2]. As with clear cell RCC, both sporadic and hereditary forms of pRCC have been described. In both sporadic and hereditary forms, pRCC may present with unifocal or bilateral and multifocal tumors. Hereditary forms of pRCC include hereditary papillary renal carcinoma (HPRC) and hereditary leiomyomatosis and renal cell carcinoma (HLRCC); papillary RCC has been seen infrequently in patients with other hereditary syndromes such as Birt-Hogg-Dubé (BHD) [4–6]. Based on various studies, a higher incidence of sporadic pRCC is thought to occur in patients with end-stage renal disease (ESRD) and acquired renal cystic disease (ARCD) compared to the general population [7, 8]. However, the risk association of ESRD with pRCC was not seen in a more recent Japanese study of over 400 patients with dialysis-associated RCC [9].

R. Srinivasan, M.D., Ph.D (✉) · K. Hammerich, M.D., Ph.D
Urologic Oncology Branch, Center for Cancer Research, National Cancer Institute, Rockville, MD, USA
e-mail: ramasrin@mail.nih.gov

© Springer Nature Switzerland AG 2019
G. G. Malouf, N. M. Tannir (eds.), *Rare Kidney Tumors*,
https://doi.org/10.1007/978-3-319-96989-3_5

5.2 Clinical Presentation

A majority of pRCCs are discovered incidentally during workup of unrelated conditions, although classic symptoms of kidney cancer such as flank pain and hematuria may be the initial presenting symptom in some. Like ccRCC, pRCC occurs more frequently in men than in women, with a ratio that ranges from 2:1 to 3.9:1. Although most pRCCs present with unilateral tumors, pRCC is most likely of all renal tumors to be associated with bilaterality and/or multifocality [1]. In inherited forms of RCC such as HLRCC, other clinical sequelae of the disease, such as the presence of cutaneous or uterine leiomyomas, may be the presenting symptom and, in the appropriate clinical setting, should prompt further evaluation. Although both ccRCC and at least some pRCC are believed to originate from the proximal tubule, they are morphologically and genetically discrete malignancies and are characterized by disparate clinical behavior. Many pRCCs, particularly papillary type 1 variants, are confined to the kidney and are associated with a favorable prognosis. However, higher-stage tumors are more likely to recur and/or metastasize. As is the case with other forms of RCC, higher-grade nuclear features and sarcomatoid differentiation are associated with worse prognosis.

5.3 Imaging Findings

Most RCCs are incidentally diagnosed at imaging; the number of cases diagnosed by the classic triad of hematuria, flank pain, and a mass in the abdomen continues to decline. While the majority of renal masses can be identified by ultrasound, magnetic resonance imaging (MRI) and high-resolution computed tomography (CT) remain the gold standard for characterizing renal masses [10]. In general, renal masses can be classified on the basis of their CT/MRI appearance as solid or cystic masses. Solid tumors can appear homogeneous and uniform or heterogeneous, with areas of necrosis. A majority of solid enhancing renal masses found at imaging represent a malignant renal tumor, with benign entities such as oncocytomas and lipid-poor angiomyolipomas being less common. Generally, pRCC is more likely to be homogeneous compared to ccRCC in CT imaging studies, particularly when the tumors are small (<3 cm in diameter). However, pRCCs larger than 3 cm in diameter may be heterogeneous with areas of necrosis and hemorrhage [11, 12]. Although there is no large study that compares differences in imaging characteristics between type 1 and type 2 pRCCs, type 2 pRCC has been described as heterogeneous with necrotic areas and indistinct borders, while type 1 pRCC is more likely to present as smaller, homogenous masses [13]. Additionally, type 1 tumors often appear as hypo-enhancing masses on CT, with contrast enhancement of 10–20 Hounsfield Units and can sometimes be mistaken for renal cysts.

Although CT has traditionally been the preferred imaging study for initial evaluation of renal masses, MRI might be helpful in discerning more subtle radiographic features, especially in small renal lesions, with studies suggesting that MRI might be helpful in distinguishing between ccRCC and pRCC [14]. In the scenario where a cyst possesses pseudoenhancement or when dealing with small renal masses, additional imaging modalities such as MRI can provide useful information [15]. In a study that evaluated the characteristics of small pRCC tumors (<3 cm) on contrast enhanced MRI, the authors found several features that may help differentiate pRCC and ccRCC [14]. pRCC was frequently characterized by low signal intensity on both T1- and T2-weighted images and often displayed a pseudocapsule. In contrast, ccRCC often demonstrated a higher intensity signal on T2-weighted MRI images. Furthermore, pRCC often exhibited a homogenous pattern on T2-weighted images, whereas ccRCC displayed a hyperintense, heterogeneous pattern. When compared to CT, less post-contrast enhancement was observed in pRCC on MRI, compared to ccRCC [16, 17]. These differences in enhancement peak in the corticomedullary phase [12]. The degree of enhancement of RCC was directly proportional to the microvessel density (a measure of tumor vascularity) of the tumor [18–20].

5.4 Histopathology

Grossly, most pRCCs are cortical based and well circumscribed. The cut surface is typically a thin pale tan to brown color, and friable papillary structures may be evident. Some pRCCs may demonstrate hemorrhage, necrosis, and/or cystic degeneration. The current histologic classification of renal tumors recognizes two subtypes of pRCC—type 1 and type 2—that are characterized by differences in clinical features and outcomes and are genetically distinct. Type 1 tumors have papillae covered by a single layer of cuboidal or low columnar cells with scanty cytoplasm and low-grade nuclei. Type 2 tumors are of a higher nuclear grade and demonstrate more than one layer of cells or pseudostratification with abundant eosinophilic cytoplasm. Sarcomatoid dedifferentiation is seen in approximately 5% of pRCCs; both type 1 and type 2 tumors can demonstrate sarcomatoid differentiation, and this feature is associated with a worse prognosis [3, 21].

5.5 Genetic and Molecular Characteristics

Chromosomal alterations, such as gain of chromosomes 7 and 17, have long been known to be associated with pRCC [22]. In the late 1990s and early 2000s, evaluation of families with inherited forms of pRCC was instrumental in identifying specific genetic alterations in pRCC, exemplified by activating *MET* mutations and inactivating mutations/deletions in the *Fumarate Hydratase* gene in the germ line of HPRC and HLRCC patients, respectively [23, 24]. Subsequently, somatic mutations in *MET* were identified in a small subset of sporadic pRCC tumors; however, the genetic drivers in most pRCC tumors were unknown [25]. With the advent of more sophisticated genetic and molecular techniques, at least two large studies have performed integrated molecular profiling using multiple platforms to interrogate primary pRCC tumors at the DNA, RNA, and protein levels [2, 26]. One of these studies, coordinated by The Cancer Genome Atlas, reported findings from a series of 161 primary papillary RCCs including 75 patients with type 1 tumors, 60 with type 2 tumors, and 26 cases in which the tumor could not be characterized as either type 1 or type 2 [2]. Based on composite molecular signatures, at least four distinct papillary subgroups were identified in this study. Tumors in the C1 subgroup, comprised largely of type 1 tumors, were associated with the best outcomes. Tumors in this subgroup were characterized by gain of chromosomes 7 and 17, as well as alterations in *MET* (activating mutations, splice variants, as well as gene fusions) that would be predicted to activate the Met pathway.

Subgroups C2a, C2b, and C2c were comprised largely of type 2 tumors and were associated with different outcomes. The C2a molecular group consisted of early-stage tumors with outcomes similar to that seen with C1 tumors, while C2b included later-stage tumors, had an intermediate prognosis, and was characterized by the presence of mutations in *SETD2*. C2c had the poorest survival and was associated with a CpG island methylator phenotype, exemplified by fumarate hydratase-deficient tumors. Other recurring alterations in type 2 pRCC included loss of CDKN2A, activation of the NRF2 oxidative stress response pathway, mutations of *FH*, gene fusions involving the MiTF gene family members TFE3 and TFEB, and mutations in chromatin remodeling genes.

5.6   Inherited Forms of pRCC

Although 5–8% of all renal tumors are believed to be inherited, the true incidence of hereditary pRCC is unknown [27]. The prevalence of some familial variants is probably an underestimation; the recent recognition of distinct forms of inherited pRCC as well as greater awareness of features associated with these entities is likely to lead to an increase in the proportion of these tumors. Hereditary RCC is characterized by early age of onset and often presents with bilateral and/or multifocal renal tumors, a positive family history of RCC, associated findings (such as skin or uterine leiomyomas in HLRCC), and often distinct histologic characteristics [2, 27]. A detailed personal, surgical, and family history and careful physical exam are essential in this patient population. Features suggestive of hereditary RCC should prompt counseling and evaluation for appropriate germ line genetic testing. The risk of multiple surgical procedures, resultant nephron loss, and subsequent development of chronic kidney disease is very high in patients with inherited forms of pRCC; additionally, clinical decision-making in these patients can be challenging, and there are special considerations in the management of conditions such as HLRCC. Owing to these unique challenges, a multidisciplinary approach to management is recommended to optimize clinical care in these patients. HPRC and HLRCC are the two best studied forms of familial pRCC, although pRCC may also be seen in BHD and other familial RCC syndromes.

5.7   HPRC

Hereditary papillary renal cell carcinoma (HPRC) was first described in 1994 by Zbar et al. [28]. Physicians managing patients with HPRC are faced with a unique set of challenges: These patients are at risk for developing over 3000 tumors in each kidney and may require multiple surgical procedures, increasing the risk for development of CKD. To date, renal tumors are the only known clinical manifestation of HPRC. Patients with disease confined to the kidneys are generally managed surgically. The primary goal of surgical treatment in HPRC patients (and other patients with bilateral multifocal tumors) is to prevent metastasis while maximizing renal preservation and delaying dialysis [29–32]. Patients with HPRC should be followed closely with abdominal imaging, and a partial nephrectomy is typically recommended when the largest tumor is greater than 3 cm. This entity shows an autosomal dominant inheritance pattern and is highly penetrant with an average age of onset of renal manifestations in the sixth decade. However, Schmidt et al. described an early-onset form where the median age of presentation was 46, with cases known to present as early as the third decade of life [33]. Individuals who are affected with HPRC have a germ line gain of function or activating mutation in the tyrosine kinase (TK) domain of the *MET* proto-oncogene, located on chromosome 7q [34]. Mutations in the TK domain of *MET* lead to constitutive activation of the Met pathway, believed to play a key role in tumorigenesis. Additionally, tumors from HPRC patients demonstrate gain of chromosome 7, resulting from nonrandom duplication of the chromosome bearing the mutant *MET* allele [23].

Renal tumors associated with HPRC are morphologically consistent with type 1 pRCC and usually exhibit low nuclear grade. Focal areas of clear cells with intracytoplasmic lipid and glycogen were also present in up to 94% of tumors from HPRC patients in one study. However, these tumors can be distinguished from conventional ccRCC tumors by the presence of small basophilic nuclei and the lack of a fine vascular network. Type 1 pRCC tumors are characterized by the presence of foamy macrophages in fibrovascular cores [35]. Kidneys of patients with HPRC often show multiple macroscopic and microscopic lesions, ranging from tumors that are less than the size of a single tubule to papillary adenoma (<0.5 cm) and to pRCC (>0.5 cm) [35]. It is estimated that 1100–3400 papillary tumors are present in a single kidney in patients with HPRC [31].

5.8   HLRCC

HLRCC was first described as a distinct entity in 2001. HLRCC is inherited in an autosomal dominant fashion and linked to mutations in a gene on chromosome 1q that was subsequently identified as the *fumarate hydratase* gene [24]. The clinical manifestations of HLRCC include cutaneous and uterine leiomyomas as well as an aggressive type 2 pRCC variant [24, 36]. Cutaneous leiomyomas are often asymptomatic but can be associated with pain. Uterine leiomyomas are generally multiple, are characterized by an early age of onset, and are usually symptomatic, requiring surgical intervention as early as the third decade of life. While leiomyomas are highly penetrant, with >90% of affected women likely to develop uterine leiomyomas in their lifetime, it is estimated that only 15–30% of affected individuals will develop a renal tumor [36–38]. Most patients with HLRCC-associated renal tumors present with a solitary primary although bilateral, multifocal tumors have also been described. Recently, it has been reported that approximately 7.8% of patients affected by HLRCC develop primary adrenal nodules consistent with macronodular adrenal hyperplasia [39].

Kidney cancer associated with HLRCC is clinically aggressive with a propensity for metastasis even when the primary tumors are small, and patients with HLRCC kidney cancer often present with nodal metastasis. As a result, early intervention when any solid renal masses are discovered is critical. HLRCC-associated kidney cancer presents several unique surgical challenges: small cysts may contain a lining infiltrated with tumor cells that are not easily seen with conventional imaging, tumors can be difficult to find on intraoperative ultrasound, borders of the tumor are often ill-defined and irregular, and spillage of HLRCC tumor often results in seeding of tumor in the peritoneum or retroperitoneum [40, 41].

Histopathological analysis of HLRCC-associated renal tumors generally reveals a single solid or solid-cystic mass with a prominent papillary pattern, although a variety of architectural patterns have been described. In a study of 40 HLRCC-associated renal tumors from patients with a known germ line FH mutation, 25 cases had a papillary architecture, 8 cases were tubulopapillary, 2 cases were tubular, 1 case was solid, and 4 cases demonstrated a mixed pattern [42]. Renal tumors associated with HLRCC have a characteristic appearance on histopathologic evaluation, demonstrating a large nucleus with a very prominent inclusion-like orangiophilic or eosinophilic nucleolus and a clear perinuclear halo [42].

Patients with HLRCC have a germ line inactivating mutation or deletion of *FH*, with a second, somatic alteration in renal tumors leading to loss of fumarate hydratase activity and disruption of the TCA cycle. Fumarate hydratase catalyzes the conversion of fumarate to malate in the Krebs or tricarboxylic acid (TCA) cycle [40, 43]. Disruption of the TCA cycle resulting from FH inactivation has several consequences. The efficient generation of ATP from glucose required to sustain cellular bioenergetic requirements is disrupted as is the generation of single carbon molecules required for macromolecule synthesis. In order to compensate, affected cells resort to aerobic glycolysis to generate ATP, a far less efficient process requiring a large and steady supply of glucose. This obligate metabolic shift to aerobic glycolysis, also known as the Warburg effect, was initially described in the 1920s as a hallmark of cancer cells. Inactivation of fumarate hydratase also leads to accumulation of its substrate, fumarate, which plays an important role in tumorigenesis in FH-deficient cells. One of the better understood consequences of fumarate accumulation is competitive inhibition of a group of cellular enzymes known as dioxygenases which catalyze diverse biochemical reactions including hydroxylation of proline residues on hypoxia inducible factors (HIF), a key component of the cellular oxygen sensing machinery. In the absence of prolyl hydroxylation, regulation of HIF by E3 ligase-dependent ubiquitination is disrupted, resulting in intracellular HIF accumulation and transcriptional activation of a variety of angiogenic (e.g., vascular endothelial growth factor) and tumorigenic factors as well as upregulation of molecules required for glucose transportation (e.g., GLUT 1) and other components of aerobic glycolysis [44]. Fumarate accumulation also results in posttranslational modification (succination) of a variety of proteins including KEAP1, a component of an E3 ligase that regulates NRF2, a key regulator of the cellular oxidative stress response [45, 46]. Succination of KEAP1 promotes stabilization and nuclear translocation of NRF2 and activation of several components of the stress response pathway thought to be critical in protecting the cells from oxidative stress engendered by Krebs cycle dysregulation.

5.9 Management

5.9.1 Localized or Organ-Confined Disease

Clinically, pRCC can be divided into organ-confined and metastatic disease states, with some studies showing better overall survival compared to ccRCC in localized states and worse prognosis in the metastatic state [47–49]. Localized sporadic pRCC is generally managed in a similar fashion to sporadic ccRCC [50, 51]; management options include active surveillance, nephrectomy (partial or radical, open, or minimally invasive), or ablative techniques [cryoablation, radiofrequency ablation (RFA), and microwave ablation (MWA)]. Active surveillance is a viable option in some patients who have small, slow-growing renal masses and are elderly, with significant competing comorbidity, or do not desire surgery. Patients on active surveillance are monitored via serial abdominal imaging (CT, MR, or ultrasound) with the intention of intervention if there are signs of progression during follow-up. Management recommendations for localized disease in hereditary pRCC are disease specific. The current recommendation for patients with HPRC is surveillance of small tumors, with surgical intervention when tumors approach 3 cm in size, to minimize the risk of metastatic disease. However, as described earlier, the high risk of metastases with HLRCC-associated renal tumors dictates the need for early surgical intervention in these patients.

When a partial nephrectomy is the preferred treatment of choice, nephron-sparing surgery (NSS) is generally used, particularly in type 1 variants with small primaries [51]. Renal masses ≤4 cm in size that are limited to the kidney (pT1) are generally managed surgically with NSS with very promising outcomes. However, the approach to advanced disease is less satisfactory, and the standard of care continues to evolve. Importantly, NSS is not the preferred management option in patients with HLRCC, where any residual tumor carries the risk of rapid progression and metastasis. In this patient cohort, it is important to obtain a wide margin during partial nephrectomy in order ensure that the entire tumor is removed with no positive surgical margin. Radical nephrectomy should still be considered for patients with tumors that are judged by the surgeon not to be amenable to partial nephrectomy due to location, size, body habitus, prior surgeries, or comorbidities.

5.9.2 Advanced Disease

Although a variety of targeted and immunomodulatory agents have shown activity in advanced ccRCC, there are currently no agents of proven clinical benefit for most patients with pRCC. Most VEGFR-targeted tyrosine kinase inhibitors and inhibitors of the mTOR pathway, while active in ccRCC, are associated with modest activity in pRCC [52, 53]. However, in the absence of other reasonable alternatives, early efforts to define optimal therapeutic choices in these patients focused comparing the relative efficacies of VEGFR and mTOR inhibitors. At least two randomized phase 2 studies in patients with nonclear cell RCC (including pRCC patients) comparing sunitinib to everolimus have been conducted; median PFS in both studies were in the range of 4–8 months with no clear evidence that one approach was superior to the other [54, 55]. Concomitant targeting of the VEGF and mTOR axis has also been evaluated in this patient population. Results from a single-arm phase 2 study of bevacizumab in combination with everolimus in patients with a wide array of treatment-naïve nonclear cell renal tumors were recently reported. A small number of patients with papillary features were included in this study, with 1/4 patients with papillary RCC and 6/14 patients with "unclassified RCC" with papillary features demonstrating an objective response [56].

As we begin to unravel the diverse molecular alterations underlying pRCC, it is becoming increasingly clear that pRCC is comprised of a heterogenous group of malignancies and a single treatment regimen is unlikely to be universally effective. A variety of pathway-directed strategies targeting distinct molecular alterations are currently under investigation and are beginning to demonstrate the value of a more personalized approach to the treatment of these tumors. One such approach is illustrated by a phase 2 study of the dual Met/VEGFR inhibitor foretinib [57]. Although the agent resulted in a modest response rate (overall response rate of 14%) in unselected patients with pRCC ($n = 74$), a subgroup of patients with Met-driven tumors (characterized by germ line *MET* mutations, $n = 10$) demonstrated a more notable response, with an overall response rate of 50%. Several ongoing phase 2 studies with a variety of Met-directed agents are in the process of further evaluating the utility of this approach and include built-in biomarker analyses to determine the correlation between Met activation and treatment outcome.

Metabolic alterations, particularly a reliance on aerobic glycolysis, characterize some papillary renal tumors, a feature exemplified in tumors with fumarate hydratase deficiency. An ongoing phase 2 study of bevacizumab in combination with erlotinib in patients with pRCC was designed to exploit the dependence of these tumors on aerobic glycolysis [58]. Preliminary results from this study revealed a high response rate in patients whose tumors are associated with fumarate hydratase deficiency ($n = 20$, ORR 65%) as well as in sporadic papillary RCC ($n = 21$, ORR

29%); the regimen continues to be evaluated in a larger patient cohort, and efforts are ongoing to identify specific subsets of sporadic pRCC most likely to respond to this approach.

Despite the early promise shown by some of the aforementioned approaches, there is currently no clear standard of care for pRCC patients with metastatic disease, and referral to a well-designed study remains the preferred option.

5.10 Summary

Papillary renal cell carcinoma refers to a heterogenous group of renal malignancies that are characterized histologically by a papillary or tubulopapillary morphology. pRCC is the second most common subtype of kidney cancer, accounting for approximately 15–20% of renal malignancies. pRCC can be inherited or occur sporadically. Histologically, two primary variants are recognized—type 1 and type 2 pRCC; type 2 pRCC can be further classified into at least three distinct molecular subgroups. There are two well-characterized hereditary syndromes associated with pRCC: (1) HPRC, a rare entity characterized by bilateral multifocal type 1 papillary kidney cancer, and (2) HLRCC, associated with an aggressive, type 2 papillary kidney tumor as well as uterine and cutaneous leiomyomas. Localized pRCC is best managed surgically, with nephron-sparing approaches preferred in small, low-grade renal tumors. There are currently no standard systemic therapy options for patients with advanced disease; however, better molecular characterization of individual pRCC subgroups has spawned interest in a variety of pathway-directed targeted therapy approaches that have shown early clinical promise.

References

1. Reuter VE. The pathology of renal epithelial neoplasms. Semin Oncol. 2006;33(5):534–43.
2. Cancer Genome Atlas Research Network, et al. Comprehensive molecular characterization of papillary renal-cell carcinoma. N Engl J Med. 2016;374(2):135–45.
3. Eble JN, Sauter G, Epstein JI, Sesterhenn IA. WHO classification of tumours: pathology and genetics of tumours of the urinary system and male genital organs. Paris: International Agency for Research on Cancer; 2004.
4. Linehan WM, Srinivasan R, Schmidt LS. The genetic basis of kidney cancer: a metabolic disease. Nat Rev Urol. 2010;7(5):277–85.
5. Pavlovich CP, et al. Evaluation and management of renal tumors in the Birt-Hogg-Dube syndrome. J Urol. 2005;173(5):1482–6.
6. Pavlovich CP, et al. Renal tumors in the Birt-Hogg-Dube syndrome. Am J Surg Pathol. 2002;26(12):1542–52.
7. Gontero P, et al. Prognostic factors in a prospective series of papillary renal cell carcinoma. BJU Int. 2008;102(6):697–702.
8. Ishikawa I, Kovacs G. High incidence of papillary renal cell tumours in patients on chronic haemodialysis. Histopathology. 1993;22(2):135–40.
9. Ikezawa E, et al. Clinical symptoms predict poor overall survival in chronic-dialysis patients with renal cell carcinoma associated with end-stage renal disease. Jpn J Clin Oncol. 2014;44(11):1096–100.

10. Vikram R, et al. Papillary renal cell carcinoma: radiologic-pathologic correlation and Spectrum of disease. Radiographics. 2009;29(3):741–54.
11. Herts BR, et al. Enhancement characteristics of papillary renal neoplasms revealed on triphasic helical CT of the kidneys. AJR Am J Roentgenol. 2002;178(2):367–72.
12. Kim JK, et al. Differentiation of subtypes of renal cell carcinoma on helical CT scans. AJR Am J Roentgenol. 2002;178(6):1499–506.
13. Yamada T, et al. Differentiation of pathologic subtypes of papillary renal cell carcinoma on CT. AJR Am J Roentgenol. 2008;191(5):1559–63.
14. Roy C, et al. MR imaging of papillary renal neoplasms: potential application for characterization of small renal masses. Eur Radiol. 2007;17(1):193–200.
15. Wang ZJ, et al. Renal cyst pseudoenhancement at multidetector CT: what are the effects of number of detectors and peak tube voltage? Radiology. 2008;248(3):910–6.
16. Weiss RM, et al. Angiographic appearance of renal papillary-tubular adenocarcinomas. J Urol. 1969;102(6):661–4.
17. Blath RA, Mancilla-Jimenez R, Stanley RJ. Clinical comparison between vascular and avascular renal cell carcinoma. J Urol. 1976;115(5):514–9.
18. Jinzaki M, Kuribayashi S. Dynamic contrast-enhanced CT of renal cell carcinoma for evaluation of tumor vascularity: analysis of single-phase or multiphase scanning. AJR Am J Roentgenol. 2007;188(6):W569. author reply W570
19. Wang JH, et al. Dynamic CT evaluation of tumor vascularity in renal cell carcinoma. AJR Am J Roentgenol. 2006;186(5):1423–30.
20. Jinzaki M, et al. Double-phase helical CT of small renal parenchymal neoplasms: correlation with pathologic findings and tumor angiogenesis. J Comput Assist Tomogr. 2000;24(6):835–42.
21. Delahunt B, et al. Morphologic typing of papillary renal cell carcinoma: comparison of growth kinetics and patient survival in 66 cases. Hum Pathol. 2001;32(6):590–5.
22. Balint I, et al. Trisomy 7 and 17 mark papillary renal cell tumours irrespectively of variation of the phenotype. J Clin Pathol. 2009;62(10):892–5.
23. Zhuang Z, et al. Trisomy 7-harbouring non-random duplication of the mutant MET allele in hereditary papillary renal carcinomas. Nat Genet. 1998;20(1):66–9.
24. Tomlinson IP, et al. Germline mutations in FH predispose to dominantly inherited uterine fibroids, skin leiomyomata and papillary renal cell cancer. Nat Genet. 2002;30(4):406–10.
25. Schmidt L, et al. Germline and somatic mutations in the tyrosine kinase domain of the MET proto-oncogene in papillary renal carcinomas. Nat Genet. 1997;16(1):68–73.
26. Durinck S, et al. Spectrum of diverse genomic alterations define non-clear cell renal carcinoma subtypes. Nat Genet. 2015;47(1):13–21.
27. Shuch B, et al. Defining early-onset kidney cancer: implications for germline and somatic mutation testing and clinical management. J Clin Oncol. 2014;32(5):431–7.
28. Zbar B, et al. Hereditary papillary renal cell carcinoma. J Urol. 1994;151(3):561–6.
29. Bratslavsky G, Linehan WM. Long-term management of bilateral, multifocal, recurrent renal carcinoma. Nat Rev Urol. 2010;7(5):267–75.
30. Herring JC, et al. Parenchymal sparing surgery in patients with hereditary renal cell carcinoma: 10-year experience. J Urol. 2001;165(3):777–81.
31. Ornstein DK. Prevalence of microscopic tumors in normal appearing renal parenchyma of patients with hereditary papillary renal cancer. J Urol. 2000;163:431–3.
32. Singer EA, et al. Outcomes of patients with surgically treated bilateral renal masses and a minimum of 10 years of followup. J Urol. 2012;188(6):2084–8.
33. Schmidt LS, et al. Early onset hereditary papillary renal carcinoma: germline missense mutations in the tyrosine kinase domain of the met proto-oncogene. J Urol. 2004;172(4 Pt 1):1256–61.
34. Schmidt L, et al. Two north American families with hereditary papillary renal carcinoma and identical novel mutations in the MET proto-oncogene. Cancer Res. 1998;58(8):1719–22.
35. Lubensky IA, et al. Hereditary and sporadic papillary renal carcinomas with c-met mutations share a distinct morphological phenotype. Am J Pathol. 1999;155(2):517–26.

36. Menko F, et al. Hereditary leiomyomatosis and renal cell cancer (HLRCC): renal cancer risk, surveillance and treatment. Familial Cancer. 2014;13(4):637–44.
37. Singer EA, et al. Impact of genetics on the diagnosis and treatment of renal cancer. Curr Urol Rep. 2011;12(1):47–55.
38. Linehan WM, Srinivasan R, Garcia JA. Non-clear cell renal cancer: disease-based management and opportunities for targeted therapeutic approaches. Semin Oncol. 2013;40(4):511–20.
39. Shuch B, et al. Adrenal nodular hyperplasia in hereditary leiomyomatosis and renal cell cancer. J Urol. 2013;189(2):430–5.
40. Linehan WM, Ricketts CJ. The metabolic basis of kidney cancer. Semin Cancer Biol. 2013;23(1):46–55.
41. Metwalli AR, Linehan WM. Nephron-sparing surgery for multifocal and hereditary renal tumors. Curr Opin Urol. 2014;24(5):466–73.
42. Merino MJ, et al. The morphologic spectrum of kidney tumors in hereditary leiomyomatosis and renal cell carcinoma (HLRCC) syndrome. Am J Surg Pathol. 2007;31(10):1578–85.
43. Shuch B, Linehan WM, Srinivasan R. Aerobic glycolysis: a novel target in kidney cancer. Expert Rev Anticancer Ther. 2013;13(6):711–9.
44. Isaacs JS, et al. HIF overexpression correlates with biallelic loss of fumarate hydratase in renal cancer: novel role of fumarate in regulation of HIF stability. Cancer Cell. 2005;8(2):143–53.
45. Kobayashi A, et al. Oxidative stress sensor Keap1 functions as an adaptor for Cul3-based E3 ligase to regulate proteasomal degradation of Nrf2. Mol Cell Biol. 2004;24(16):7130–9.
46. Adam J, et al. Renal cyst formation in Fh1-deficient mice is independent of the Hif/Phd pathway: roles for fumarate in KEAP1 succination and Nrf2 signaling. Cancer Cell. 2011;20(4):524–37.
47. Leibovich BC, et al. Histological subtype is an independent predictor of outcome for patients with renal cell carcinoma. J Urol. 2010;183(4):1309–16.
48. Ronnen EA, et al. Treatment outcome for metastatic papillary renal cell carcinoma patients. Cancer. 2006;107(11):2617–21.
49. Steffens S, et al. Incidence and long-term prognosis of papillary compared to clear cell renal cell carcinoma--a multicentre study. Eur J Cancer. 2012;48(15):2347–52.
50. Campbell SC, et al. Guideline for management of the clinical T1 renal mass. J Urol. 2009;182(4):1271–9.
51. Ljungberg B, et al. EAU Guidelines on Renal Cell Carcinoma: 2014 Update. Eur Urol. 2015;67(5):913–24.
52. Escudier BJ, Bracarda S, Maroto Rey JP, Szczylik C, Nathan PD, Negrier S, Cattaneo A, Weiss C, Porta C, Gruenwald V. Open-label, phase II raptor study of everolimus (EVE) for papillary mRCC: efficacy in type 1 and type 2 histology. J Clin Oncol. 2014;32(suppl 4):410.
53. Ravaud A, et al. First-line treatment with sunitinib for type 1 and type 2 locally advanced or metastatic papillary renal cell carcinoma: a phase II study (SUPAP) by the French genitourinary group (GETUG)dagger. Ann Oncol. 2015;26(6):1123–8.
54. Armstrong AJ, et al. Everolimus versus sunitinib for patients with metastatic non-clear cell renal cell carcinoma (ASPEN): a multicentre, open-label, randomised phase 2 trial. Lancet Oncol. 2016;17(3):378–88.
55. Tannir NM, et al. Everolimus versus Sunitinib prospective evaluation in metastatic non-clear cell renal cell carcinoma (ESPN): a randomized multicenter phase 2 trial. Eur Urol. 2016;69(5):866–74.
56. Voss MH, et al. Phase II trial and correlative genomic analysis of Everolimus plus Bevacizumab in advanced non-clear cell renal cell carcinoma. J Clin Oncol. 2016;34(32):3846–53.
57. Choueiri TK, et al. Phase II and biomarker study of the dual MET/VEGFR2 inhibitor foretinib in patients with papillary renal cell carcinoma. J Clin Oncol. 2013;31(2):181–6.
58. Srinivasan R, et al. Mechanism based targeted therapy for hereditary leiomyomatosis and renal cell cancer (HLRCC) and sporadic papillary renal cell carcinoma: interim results from a phase 2 study of bevacizumab and erlotinib. In: NCI-AACR-EORTC molecular targets meeting, Barcelona, 2014.

Renal Medullary Carcinoma

6

Pavlos Msaouel, Priya Rao, and Nizar M. Tannir

6.1 Introduction

First described in 1995 [1], renal medullary carcinoma (RMC) predominantly afflicts young adults and adolescents with sickle cell trait and is one of the most aggressive renal cell carcinomas [2, 3]. It arises from the renal papillae or calyceal epithelium of the renal medulla. In the original series by Davis et al. [1], the median overall survival of patients with RMC was only 4 months, and despite therapy it has only improved to 13 months in the most recent series of cases [3]. RMC is very rare, comprising <0.5% of all renal cell carcinomas [4], but its incidence is likely underestimated as it is a challenging diagnosis that can often be mistaken for collecting duct carcinoma or other aggressive kidney malignancies [5].

Similarly to other renal malignancies such as clear cell renal cell carcinoma and collecting duct carcinoma [6–8], men are twice as likely to be affected by RMC than women [3, 9]. Afflicted patients have a median age of 28 years (range 9–48 years), and most patients (~67%) will present with metastatic disease, primarily to the lymph nodes (85% of cases), lungs (46%), liver (15%), and bone (15%) [3]. Metastases to the central nervous system are extremely rare (<1% of cases) [3, 9], suggesting a low predilection of the disease to the brain parenchyma. Approximately 27% of patients with metastatic disease will have one to two metastatic sites, whereas 73% of patients will have more than two sites of metastatic involvement [3].

P. Msaouel · P. Rao · N. M. Tannir (✉)
Department of Genitourinary Medical Oncology, The University of Texas MD Anderson Cancer Center, Houston, TX, USA
e-mail: ntannir@mdanderson.org

© Springer Nature Switzerland AG 2019
G. G. Malouf, N. M. Tannir (eds.), *Rare Kidney Tumors*,
https://doi.org/10.1007/978-3-319-96989-3_6

6.2   Renal Medullary Carcinoma and Sickle Hemoglobinopathies

Although all sickle hemoglobinopathies are associated with RMC, the vast majority of patients with RMC have sickle cell trait (SCT) [3, 9], and only a handful of cases have been documented in patients with homozygous sickle cell disease [9–11], hemoglobin SC disease [9, 10], or sickle beta thalassemia [3, 9]. This may be due to the much higher population genotype rates of SCT (8.3% in the United States) compared with sickle cell disease (0.15%) [12, 13]. Approximately 1 in 14 African Americans have sickle cell trait [14], and between 1/20,000 and 1/39,000 will develop RMC [9]. SCT is found in approximately 300 million individuals worldwide [15]. The prevalence rates of SCT vary from ~7% among African Americans [14], 23.5% in the Chalkidiki peninsula of Greece [16], and 10% in the Çukurova region of Southern Turkey [17] up to 13% among some populations in Central India [18], 20% in the Eastern Province of Saudi Arabia [19], and between 10% and 40% across equatorial Africa, reaching 45% among the Baamba tribe in Uganda [20]. Nevertheless, other than the United States and Europe, RMC has very rarely, if at all, been described in these areas. This is likely due to underreporting, although the possibility of environmental or other locoregional factors contributing to a higher RMC incidence cannot be excluded. Other than the presence of sickle hemoglobinopathy, there is no known familial predisposition or environmental risk factor that can explain why only certain patients will develop RMC. Due to the enigmatic pathogenesis of RMC, no effective prevention strategies have been developed, and there is no evidence that screening of all individuals with SCT for RMC will be beneficial.

RMC is more likely to arise from the right (~70% of cases) compared with the left kidney [3, 9], a laterality that is also found in collecting duct carcinomas [5]. Notably, other renal manifestations of sickle cell trait such as hematuria predominantly arise from the left kidney due to the compression of the left renal vein between the aorta and superior mesenteric artery which causes relative anoxia in the renal medulla and thus promotes sickling, an effect known as the nutcracker phenomenon [21]. One explanation for this discrepancy in the laterality of sickle nephropathies and RMC may be that the driver of RMC pathogenesis is regional ischemia induced by red blood cell sickling in the medullary vasa recta [13]. Anatomical differences in the right vs. the left renal artery [22] may result in reduced blood flow and increased viscosity from red blood cell sickling in the right renal inner medulla [13]. Sex differences in the propensity for regional ischemia among individuals with sickle hemoglobinopathies [23, 24] may also explain why RMC is two times more frequent in men than women [3, 9, 13].

6.3   Molecular Alterations

Renal medullary carcinoma is characterized by complete loss of expression of the SMARCB1 protein (also known as INI1, hSNF5, or BAF47) [25, 26], an important subunit of the SWI/SNF complex, which hydrolyzes ATP to remodel chromatin structure, thus facilitating gene expression [27]. SMARCB1, encoded on chromosome 22q11.2, is a tumor suppressor that is frequently inactivated in a variety of adult and childhood malignancies including RMC (100% of cases), malignant rhabdoid tumors (~98%), and epithelioid sarcomas (~90%), as well as subsets of epithelioid malignant peripheral nerve sheath tumors (~50%), myoepithelial carcinomas (~40% of Paediatric cases and 10% of adult cases), and extraskeletal myxoid chondrosarcomas (~17%) [28]. Recent studies in small RMC cohorts indicate that in at least some RMC cases, loss of one or both of the *SMARCB1* alleles occurs via inactivating translocations [29, 30]. Other mechanisms by which *SMARCB1* may be inactivated include single-nucleotide deletions, inactivating nonsynonymous polymorphisms, large deletions, or monosomies. In addition to these genetic alterations, it is possible that SMARCB1 may be inactivated by epigenetic mechanisms such as methylation of the *SMARCB1* promoter or micro-ribonucleic acid (miRNA) silencing of gene expression.

Loss of SMARCB1 destabilizes, but does not completely abrogate, the SWI/SNF complex [31, 32]. Residual SMARCB1-deficient SWI/SNF complexes demonstrate altered DNA-binding patterns resulting in distinct transcriptional profiles that may promote tumorigenesis [31, 32]. Because SMARCB1 loss is seen in all RMC cases, it is likely that this alteration appears early during carcinogenesis and provides a selective growth advantage to initial tumor or tumor precursor cells. It remains to be determined whether, and which, pathways altered by SMARCB1 loss continue to drive cell growth in full-fledged RMC tumors. In malignant rhabdoid tumors, SMARCB1 loss promotes chromosomal instability and aneuploidy due to defective chromosome segregation [33]. It is possible that such events can stochastically produce genetic alterations that may drive tumor cell growth independently of the biologic pathways directly affected by SMARCB1 loss.

The SWI/SNF complex acts antagonistically to the enhancer of zeste homolog 2 (EZH2), a methyltransferase that represses gene transcription by trimethylating histone H3 on lysine 27 (H3K27me3) [34]. Increased EZH2 activity can drive tumor cell growth by repressing cell differentiation pathways [27, 34]. Accordingly, therapeutic inhibition of the histone methyltransferase activity of EZH2 promotes cell death in SMARCB1-deficient malignancies such as malignant rhabdoid tumors [35], indicating that cell growth depends on EZH2. This prompted an ongoing phase II trial (clinicaltrials.gov NCT02601950) evaluating the antitumor efficacy of tazemetostat, an inhibitor of EZH2 methyltransferase activity, in SMARB1-negative tumors such as RMC. Tazemetostat is also being tested in a phase I trial (clinicaltrials.gov NCT02601937) in Paediatric patients with relapsed or refractory SMARCB1-negative tumors. Additional oncogenic genes and pathways known to be affected by SMARCB1 loss include members of the hedgehog pathways such as Gli1 [36], the BIN1 tumor suppressor [37], the cyclin-dependent kinase inhibitor 2A pathway [38], cyclin D1 [39], and the Wnt/β-catenin pathway [40]. It remains to be determined which of these pathways, all of which were described in malignancies other than RMC, are biologically relevant and can be therapeutically targeted in RMC. Molecular profiling of RMC samples has shown increased topoisomerase IIα expression [41, 42], suggesting that these tumors may respond to topoisomerase IIα inhibitors, such as anthracyclines or podophyllotoxins. However, a recent pooled analysis of the literature was unable to detect, perhaps due to the low number of reported cases, a specific benefit from topoisomerase IIα inhibitors compared with other cytotoxic chemotherapy agents in patients with RMC [2].

Patients with SCT may also develop another distinct malignancy characterized by *anaplastic lymphoma kinase (ALK)* translocation resulting in its fusion with *vinculin (VCL)* [43]. This extremely rare *VCL-ALK* fusion renal cell carcinoma variant arises from the renal medulla of children (mean age 9 years old) with SCT and demonstrates intact *SMARCB1* expression as well as much lower proliferative activity (Ki-67 of ~5%) compared with the very high mitotic rates of SMARCB1-negative RMC. The biologic relationship between these two malignancies is not currently understood, but they may share the same pathogenetic trigger induced by red blood cell sickling in the renal medulla [13].

6.4 Diagnosis

RMC occurs in young patients (<50 years old) with SCT who most commonly present with hematuria and/or flank pain in ~66% cases, and about half will have constitutional symptoms such as unintentional weight loss or, less commonly, night sweats [3]. Histologically, RMC presents as a high-grade, poorly differentiated adenocarcinoma (Fig. 6.1) containing focal anastomosing tubules and cords with a reticular and cribriform appearance, as well as a myxoid highly desmoplastic stroma with neutrophil infiltrates and microabscess-like foci (Fig. 6.2) [1, 5]. Sickle red blood cells in the tumor specimen confirm the diagnosis (Fig. 6.3). Immunohistochemistry demonstrates loss of SMARCB1 and, in many cases,

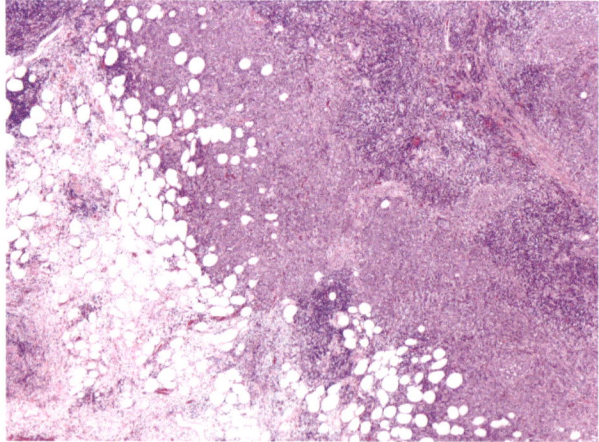

Fig. 6.1 Renal medullary carcinoma often shows widespread involvement of the perirenal soft tissue and is of a high pathologic stage at presentation. Tumor cells are usually arranged in sheets and show an ill-defined border

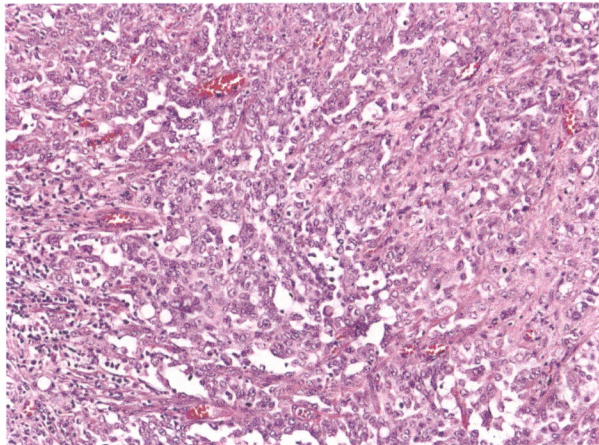

Fig. 6.2 Renal medullary carcinoma cells are of high nuclear grade and may be present in sheets, nests, or glands

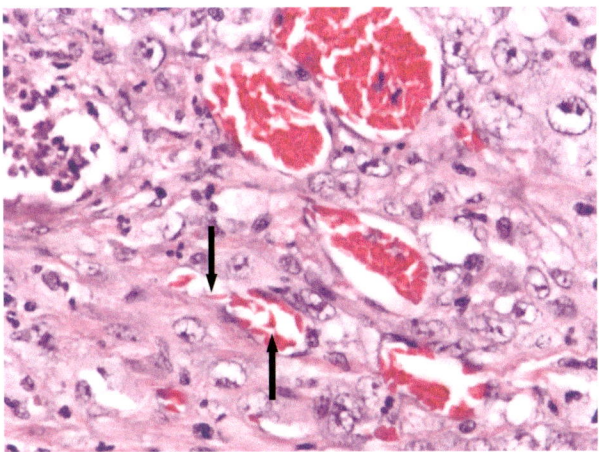

Fig. 6.3 Drepanocytes (sickle cells) may be seen in the vascular spaces of nephrectomy samples from patients with renal medullary carcinoma

expression of the stem cell marker OCT3/4 [44]. Computed tomography (CT) imaging at presentation will demonstrate an ill-defined heterogeneous mass, arising from the renal medulla, more frequently in the right kidney, with intratumoral necrosis, an average size of 6–7 cm [3], and lower contrast enhancement than the renal cortex and medulla during all phases [45].

Many of the regions where SCT is highly prevalent lack the pathology expertise or access to the special staining assays that facilitate the diagnosis of RMC. This may result in considerable underreporting of the disease. RMC should be part of the differential diagnosis in all young patients with sickle cell hemoglobinopathy who present with a renal cell carcinoma. It is particularly important to distinguish RMC from other kidney malignancies because RMC is refractory to targeted therapies that are effective in clear cell renal cell carcinoma or other non-clear cell renal cell carcinomas. The histologic and clinical similarities between RMC and collecting duct carcinoma may also pose diagnostic difficulties [5]. Because SMARCB1 loss can be seen in other malignancies [28, 46], absence of SMARCB1 expression cannot on its own be the defining characteristic of RMC. On the other hand, intact SMARCB1 nuclear expression by immunohistochemistry should exclude the diagnosis of RMC in all cases [47]. The major difference between collecting duct carcinoma and RMC is that the latter occurs only in patients with a sickle cell hemoglobinopathy. Therefore, a diagnosis of RMC can be made on the basis of appropriate histological findings (including loss of *SMARCB1* expression) in patients with sickle cell hemoglobinopathy. Furthermore, it has been proposed that patients with no evidence of hemoglobinopathy who present with high-grade renal adenocarcinomas with loss of *SMARCB1* expression (and/or presence of *OCT3/4* expression) should be diagnosed with "unclassified renal cell carcinoma with medullary phenotype" [5].

6.5   Management of Renal Medullary Carcinoma

Localized or locally advanced (stage I–III per the staging system used in clear cell renal cell carcinoma) RMC is preferably treated with nephrectomy and retroperitoneal lymph node dissection followed by close surveillance [3]. Radical nephrectomy is favored over partial nephrectomy even in very early-stage tumors due to the infiltrative nature and medullary epicenter of RMC [47]. In patients with metastatic disease, retrospective data suggest that cytoreductive nephrectomy, when feasible, results in improved overall survival (16.4 months vs. 7.0 months) compared with systemic chemotherapy alone regardless of ECOG performance status (0–1 or 2–3) or whether systemic chemotherapy is first given preoperatively or after nephrectomy [3]. Based on these data, as well as expert opinion [47], it is currently recommended that patients with locally advanced or metastatic RMC and ECOG performance status of 0–1 undergo up-front systemic chemotherapy followed by cytoreductive nephrectomy with retroperitoneal lymph node dissection, particularly if this will remove most of the tumor burden, followed by systemic chemotherapy. If the patient presents with ECOG performance status of 2–3 and/or heavy metastatic disease burden outside the primary tumor, then up-front systemic chemotherapy is again preferred and can later be followed by cytoreductive nephrectomy with retroperitoneal lymph node dissection provided there is a good response to systemic therapy. Because RMC often aggressively recurs while patients with seemingly early stage disease are still recovering from nephrectomy, up-front systemic chemotherapy should be considered for the majority of patients, irrespective of disease stage. Distant metastasectomy is generally not recommended.

   RMC is resistant to targeted antiangiogenic therapies, such as sorafenib, sunitinib, pazopanib, and bevacizumab, or mechanistic target of rapamycin (mTOR) inhibitors such as everolimus that are used against other renal cell carcinomas [3]. Therefore, these therapies should not be routinely used, outside of well-designed clinical trials, in patients with RMC. One patient with RMC treated with the proteasome inhibitor bortezomib achieved a complete response without evidence of disease recurrence for more than 2 years [48]. This patient was subsequently lost to follow-up, and since that time, no other patients with RMC have shown a response to single-agent bortezomib [49], although durable responses have been noted when it is used in combination with platinum-based chemotherapy agents followed by single-agent bortezomib maintenance [50]. A phase II clinical trial (clinicaltrials. gov NCT03587662) is evaluating the combination of the second-generation proteasome inhibitor ixazomib with gemcitabine and doxorubicin in patients with RMC. Other targeted therapies such as imatinib have not shown efficacy against RMC [3]. Newer targeted agents such as cabozantinib and lenvatinib have more recently been approved for use in clear cell renal cell carcinoma [51, 52]. There is currently no published experience with these drugs against RMC.

Cytotoxic combination chemotherapy is the only systemic treatment approach that has consistently shown to produce partial or complete responses in approximately 29% of cases [3]. Therefore, outside of clinical trials, cytotoxic combination chemotherapy remains the mainstay of systemic treatment for RMC. Unfortunately, responses are not durable in most cases, and there are no direct comparisons between the different chemotherapy regimens. Most series have used various combinations of platinum agents, taxanes, anthracyclines, or gemcitabine [2, 3]. High-dose-intensity combination of methotrexate, vinblastine, doxorubicin, and cisplatin (MVAC), commonly used in patients with urothelial cell carcinomas, has shown efficacy against RMC [49]. However, a retrospective analysis did not reveal a benefit of MVAC compared with a regimen containing cisplatin, paclitaxel, and gemcitabine (CPG) [2]. The preferred initial regimen in our institution is paclitaxel 175 mg/m^2 plus carboplatin at an area under the time-concentration curve (AUC) of six administered every 21 days. We prefer carboplatin to cisplatin to minimize nephrotoxicity in anticipation of cytoreductive nephrectomy for those patients that will respond to the systemic treatment. For second-line therapy, we choose to use agents that the patient has not previously been exposed to such as gemcitabine and doxorubicin.

Despite systemic chemotherapy, very few patients will live for >24 months [3]. Novel therapeutic strategies are therefore urgently needed. As detailed above, the EZH2 inhibitor tazemetostat is being tested in two clinical trials in adults (clinicaltrials.gov NCT02601950) and children (clinicaltrials.gov NCT02601937) with SMARCB1-deficient tumors, including RMC. Molecular analyses of tissue samples, as well as the development of in vitro and in vivo animal models of RMC, will provide further insights into the biology of this disease and help identify pathways amenable to targeted therapeutic strategies. In addition, the last few years have been marked by significant progress in the development of immune checkpoint inhibitors that can harness the immune system to target cancer cells. Programmed cell death protein 1 (PD-1) was the first immune checkpoint receptor to be targeted in clinical practice against metastatic clear cell renal carcinomas [53]. A gratifying clinical response was subsequently noted in a case report of a patient with RMC treated with nivolumab, an anti-PD-1 immune checkpoint inhibitor [54]. Analysis of this patient's tumor tissue prior to initiating nivolumab treatment revealed a robust immune infiltrate with high percentage of CD4+ and CD8+ T lymphocytes as well as robust levels of PD-L1 and PD-1 expression [54]. There is currently one active phase II clinical trial (clinicaltrials.gov NCT03274258) evaluating the efficacy of immunomodulatory agents in RMC.

6.6   Media Advocacy and Scientific Collaborations

RMC is very rare and targets particularly vulnerable populations as most patients in the United States are young, are often uninsured, and are predominantly African American. Strong media advocacy is therefore quintessential to improve awareness and communication among both patients and healthcare providers. This can facilitate the early referral, diagnosis, and management of RMC, as well as promote clinical and translational research to better understand and treat this deadly disease. Social media sites dedicated to increasing RMC awareness include http://www.rmc-support.org/ and http://chrisjohnsonfoundation.org/. To promote scientific communication and collaboration, an RMC Working Group met in April 2016 and developed consensus statements on the diagnosis and management of RMC [47]. This group also aims to develop an International Registry of patients with RMC and sickle cell hemoglobinopathies to better understand the incidence and natural history of this disease across different populations.

Conclusions

RMC is a rare and highly aggressive malignancy that predominantly affects young patients and has near universal fatality despite therapy. The association with sickle cell hemoglobinopathies, mainly sickle cell trait, is a defining feature of this disease. Although loss of the SMARCB1 protein is not an exclusive characteristic of RMC, it can be used to support the diagnosis. RMC is refractory to mTOR inhibitors and antiangiogenic agents approved for clear cell renal cell carcinoma, and responses to cytotoxic chemotherapy are typically brief. Novel treatment approaches are clearly needed for this deadly disease, and numerous questions remain unanswered regarding its prevalence, risk factors, and pathogenesis. Data from in vitro and in vivo models, integrated with the genomic, epigenomic, transcriptomic, and proteomic landscapes of RMC tumor samples, will lay the biological foundation required to identify pathways amenable to targeted or immunomodulatory therapies. Large-scale collaborative efforts will be required to characterize the global burden and natural history of RMC across different populations and to facilitate patient accrual in well-designed clinical trials.

References

1. Davis CJ Jr, Mostofi FK, Sesterhenn IA. Renal medullary carcinoma. The seventh sickle cell nephropathy. Am J Surg Pathol. 1995;19:1–11.
2. Iacovelli R, Modica D, Palazzo A, Trenta P, Piesco G, Cortesi E. Clinical outcome and prognostic factors in renal medullary carcinoma: a pooled analysis from 18 years of medical literature. Can Urol Assoc J. 2015;9:E172–7.
3. Shah AY, Karam JA, Malouf GG, et al. Management and outcomes of patients with renal medullary carcinoma: a multicentre collaborative study. BJU Int. 2017;120:782–92.
4. Shuch B, Amin A, Armstrong AJ, et al. Understanding pathologic variants of renal cell carcinoma: distilling therapeutic opportunities from biologic complexity. Eur Urol. 2015;67:85–97.
5. Amin MB, Smith SC, Agaimy A, et al. Collecting duct carcinoma versus renal medullary carcinoma: an appeal for nosologic and biological clarity. Am J Surg Pathol. 2014;38:871–4.
6. Siegel RL, Miller KD, Jemal A. Cancer statistics, 2016. CA Cancer J Clin. 2016;66:7–30.
7. Wright JL, Risk MC, Hotaling J, Lin DW. Effect of collecting duct histology on renal cell cancer outcome. J Urol. 2009;182:2595–9.
8. Tokuda N, Naito S, Matsuzaki O, et al. Collecting duct (Bellini duct) renal cell carcinoma: a nationwide survey in Japan. J Urol. 2006;176:40–3. discussion 3
9. Alvarez O, Rodriguez MM, Jordan L, Sarnaik S. Renal medullary carcinoma and sickle cell trait: a systematic review. Pediatr Blood Cancer. 2015;62:1694–9.
10. Dimashkieh H, Choe J, Mutema G. Renal medullary carcinoma: a report of 2 cases and review of the literature. Arch Pathol Lab Med. 2003;127:e135–8.
11. Marsh A, Golden C, Hoppe C, Quirolo K, Vichinsky E. Renal medullary carcinoma in an adolescent with sickle cell anemia. Pediatr Blood Cancer. 2014;61:567.
12. Bunn H, Forget B. Hemoglobin: molecular genetic and clinical aspects. Philadelphia: W. B. Saunders Company; 1986. p. 690.
13. Msaouel P, Tannir NM, Walker CL. A model linking sickle cell hemoglobinopathies and smarcb1 loss in renal medullary carcinoma. Clin Cancer Res. 2018;24(9):2044–9.
14. Ojodu J, Hulihan MM, Pope SN, Grant AM. Centers for disease C, prevention. Incidence of sickle cell trait--United States, 2010. MMWR Morb Mortal Wkly Rep. 2014;63:1155–8.
15. Grant AM, Parker CS, Jordan LB, et al. Public health implications of sickle cell trait: a report of the CDC meeting. Am J Prev Med. 2011;41:S435–9.
16. Barnicot NA, Allison AC, Blumberg BS, Deliyannis G, Krimbas C, Ballas A. Haemoglobin types in Greek populations. Ann Hum Genet. 1963;26:229–36.
17. Curuk MA, Zeren F, Genc A, Ozavci-Aygun S, Kilinc Y, Aksoy K. Prenatal diagnosis of sickle cell anemia and beta-thalassemia in southern Turkey. Hemoglobin. 2008;32:525–30.
18. Shrikhande AV, Arjunan A, Agarwal A, et al. Prevalence of the beta(S) gene among scheduled castes, scheduled tribes and other backward class groups in Central India. Hemoglobin. 2014;38:230–5.
19. Salamah MM, Mallouh AA, Hamdan JA. Acute splenic sequestration crises in Saudi children with sickle cell disease. Ann Trop Paediatr. 1989;9:115–7.
20. Sickle-cell anaemia: report by the Secretariat. 59th world health assembly, 2 April 2006.
21. Abbud-Filho M. Comments on renal abnormalities of sickle cell disease. Rev Bras Hematol Hemoter. 2013;35:311–2.
22. Merklin R, Michels N. The variant renal and suprarenal blood supply with data on the interior phrenic, ureteral and gonadal arteries: a statistical analysis based on 185 dissections and a review of the literature. J Int Coll Surg. 1958:41–76.
23. Gladwin MT, Schechter AN, Ognibene FP, et al. Divergent nitric oxide bioavailability in men and women with sickle cell disease. Circulation. 2003;107:271–8.
24. Platt OS, Brambilla DJ, Rosse WF, et al. Mortality in sickle cell disease. Life expectancy and risk factors for early death. N Engl J Med. 1994;330:1639–44.
25. Margol AS, Judkins AR. Pathology and diagnosis of SMARCB1-deficient tumors. Cancer Genet. 2014;207:358–64.

26. Cheng JX, Tretiakova M, Gong C, Mandal S, Krausz T, Taxy JB. Renal medullary carcinoma: rhabdoid features and the absence of INI1 expression as markers of aggressive behavior. Mod Pathol. 2008;21:647–52.
27. Kadoch C, Crabtree GR. Mammalian SWI/SNF chromatin remodeling complexes and cancer: mechanistic insights gained from human genomics. Sci Adv. 2015;1:e1500447.
28. Hollmann TJ, Hornick JL. INI1-deficient tumors: diagnostic features and molecular genetics. Am J Surg Pathol. 2011;35:e47–63.
29. Calderaro J, Masliah-Planchon J, Richer W, et al. Balanced translocations disrupting SMARCB1 are Hallmark recurrent genetic alterations in renal medullary carcinomas. Eur Urol. 2016;69:1055–61.
30. Carlo M, Chen Y, Chaim J, et al. Medullary renal cell carcinoma (RCC): genomics and treatment outcomes. J Clin Oncol. 2016;34:4556. suppl; abstr 4556
31. Wang X, Sansam CG, Thom CS, et al. Oncogenesis caused by loss of the SNF5 tumor suppressor is dependent on activity of BRG1, the ATPase of the SWI/SNF chromatin remodeling complex. Cancer Res. 2009;69:8094–101.
32. Wang X, Lee RS, Alver BH, et al. SMARCB1-mediated SWI/SNF complex function is essential for enhancer regulation. Nat Genet. 2017;49(2):289–95.
33. Vries RG, Bezrookove V, Zuijderduijn LM, et al. Cancer-associated mutations in chromatin remodeler hSNF5 promote chromosomal instability by compromising the mitotic checkpoint. Genes Dev. 2005;19:665–70.
34. Kim KH, Roberts CW. Targeting EZH2 in cancer. Nat Med. 2016;22:128–34.
35. Knutson SK, Warholic NM, Wigle TJ, et al. Durable tumor regression in genetically altered malignant rhabdoid tumors by inhibition of methyltransferase EZH2. Proc Natl Acad Sci U S A. 2013;110:7922–7.
36. Jagani Z, Mora-Blanco EL, Sansam CG, et al. Loss of the tumor suppressor Snf5 leads to aberrant activation of the hedgehog-Gli pathway. Nat Med. 2010;16:1429–33.
37. McKenna ES, Tamayo P, Cho YJ, et al. Epigenetic inactivation of the tumor suppressor BIN1 drives proliferation of SNF5-deficient tumors. Cell Cycle. 2012;11:1956–65.
38. Wilson BG, Wang X, Shen X, et al. Epigenetic antagonism between polycomb and SWI/SNF complexes during oncogenic transformation. Cancer Cell. 2010;18:316–28.
39. Tsikitis M, Zhang Z, Edelman W, Zagzag D, Kalpana GV. Genetic ablation of Cyclin D1 abrogates genesis of rhabdoid tumors resulting from Ini1 loss. Proc Natl Acad Sci U S A. 2005;102:12129–34.
40. Mora-Blanco EL, Mishina Y, Tillman EJ, et al. Activation of beta-catenin/TCF targets following loss of the tumor suppressor SNF5. Oncogene. 2014;33:933–8.
41. Schaeffer EM, Guzzo TJ, Furge KA, et al. Renal medullary carcinoma: molecular, pathological and clinical evidence for treatment with topoisomerase-inhibiting therapy. BJU Int. 2010;106:62–5.
42. Albadine R, Wang W, Brownlee NA, et al. Topoisomerase II alpha status in renal medullary carcinoma: immuno-expression and gene copy alterations of a potential target of therapy. J Urol. 2009;182:735–40.
43. Smith NE, Deyrup AT, Marino-Enriquez A, et al. VCL-ALK renal cell carcinoma in children with sickle-cell trait: the eighth sickle-cell nephropathy? Am J Surg Pathol. 2014;38:858–63.
44. Rao P, Tannir NM, Tamboli P. Expression of OCT3/4 in renal medullary carcinoma represents a potential diagnostic pitfall. Am J Surg Pathol. 2012;36:583–8.
45. Shi Z, Zhuang Q, You R, Li Y, Li J, Cao D. Clinical and computed tomography imaging features of renal medullary carcinoma: a report of six cases. Oncol Lett. 2016;11:261–6.
46. Elwood H, Chaux A, Schultz L, et al. Immunohistochemical analysis of SMARCB1/INI-1 expression in collecting duct carcinoma. Urology. 2011;78:474 e1–5.
47. Beckermann KE, Sharma D, Chaturvedi S, et al. Renal medullary carcinoma: establishing standards in practice. J Oncol Pract. 2017;13:414–21.
48. Ronnen EA, Kondagunta GV, Motzer RJ. Medullary renal cell carcinoma and response to therapy with Bortezomib. J Clin Oncol. 2006;24:e14.

49. Rathmell WK, Monk JP. High-dose-intensity MVAC for advanced renal medullary carcinoma: report of three cases and literature review. Urology. 2008;72:659–63.
50. Carden MA, Smith S, Meany H, Yin H, Alazraki A, Rapkin LB. Platinum plus bortezomib for the treatment of pediatric renal medullary carcinoma: two cases. Pediatr Blood Cancer. 2017;64:7.
51. Choueiri TK, Escudier B, Powles T, et al. Cabozantinib versus everolimus in advanced renal-cell carcinoma. N Engl J Med. 2015;373:1814–23.
52. Motzer RJ, Hutson TE, Glen H, et al. Lenvatinib, everolimus, and the combination in patients with metastatic renal cell carcinoma: a randomised, phase 2, open-label, multicentre trial. Lancet Oncol. 2015;16:1473–82.
53. Motzer RJ, Escudier B, McDermott DF, et al. Nivolumab versus everolimus in advanced renal-cell carcinoma. N Engl J Med. 2015;373:1803–13.
54. Beckermann KE, Jolly PC, Kim JY, et al. Clinical and immunologic correlates of response to PD-1 blockade in a patient with metastatic renal medullary carcinoma. J Immunother Cancer. 2017;5(1)

Collecting Duct Carcinoma

7

Hendrik Van Poppel, Evelyne Lerut, Raymond Oyen,
Maria Debiec-Rychter, Herlinde Dumez, Maarten Albersen,
and Steven Joniau

7.1 Introduction

Collecting duct carcinoma (CDC) of the kidney is a rare variant of renal cell carcinoma (RCC) with an extremely poor prognosis as most cases are metastatic at the time of diagnosis. RCC is a clinically, histologically and genetically heterogeneous group of tumours. The different subtypes of RCC are classified according to the cells of origin in the different parts of the nephron. Conventional (clear cell) RCC and papillary RCC show alterations linked to the proximal tubules, while chromophobe RCC and CDC are presumed to originate from the collecting duct epithelium (intercalated cells and principal cells of the collecting ducts, respectively). The collecting ducts in the kidney are also known as the Bellini's ducts, named after the Italian physician Lorenzo Bellini (1643–1704) who described these tubes for the first time (ref: https://www.britannica.com/biography/Lorenzo-Bellini). This explains why CDC is also known as Bellini duct carcinoma. Of all renal neoplasms, CDC is the most aggressive with no established treatment guidelines [1, 2].

H. Van Poppel (✉) · M. Albersen · S. Joniau
Department of Urology, University Hospitals, KU Leuven, Leuven, Belgium
e-mail: hendrik.vanpoppel@uzleuven.be

E. Lerut
Department of Pathology, University Hospitals, KU Leuven, Leuven, Belgium

R. Oyen
Department of Radiology, University Hospitals, KU Leuven, Leuven, Belgium

M. Debiec-Rychter
Department of Genetics, University Hospitals, KU Leuven, Leuven, Belgium

H. Dumez
Department of Medical Oncology, University Hospitals, KU Leuven, Leuven, Belgium

© Springer Nature Switzerland AG 2019
G. G. Malouf, N. M. Tannir (eds.), *Rare Kidney Tumors*,
https://doi.org/10.1007/978-3-319-96989-3_7

7.2 Recognition as a Unique Pathological Subtype of RCC

In 1976, Mancilla-Jimenez and colleagues first observed the atypical hyperplastic changes of adjacent collecting duct epithelium in 3 out of 34 cases of papillary RCC. The authors suggested that some papillary RCC may arise from the epithelium of the collecting ducts [3]. Since 1986, CDC is recognized as a new separate entity [4, 5]. In 1997, the Heidelberg classification of renal tumours identified five histologic types of RCC: conventional (clear cell), papillary, chromophobe, collecting duct and unclassifiable [1, 6]. In the 2004 World Health Organization (WHO) classification, CDC was also recognized as a distinct entity from conventional, papillary and chromophobe RCC [7]. Recently, new subtypes of RCC have been described: hereditary leiomyomatosis and RCC, syndrome-associated RCC, succinate dehydrogenase-deficient RCC, tubulocystic RCC, acquired cystic disease-associated RCC and clear cell papillary RCC [8, 9]. Each type has distinct histological (light and electron microscopy), immunohistochemical and cytogenetic features [9].

7.3 Epidemiology

CDC is a rare tumour of the kidney that accounts for 1–3% of all renal neoplasms [10–16]. It occurs at almost any age (range, 13–83 years) with a mean age of 55 years and predominantly affecting males (male to female ratio is 2:1) [17]. A retrospective study using the Surveillance, Epidemiology, and End Results (SEER) cases from 1973 to 2004 identified 98 patients with CDC. According to this study, 63.3% of these patients are white, 27.5% are African American and 9.2% are other races [18]. A total of 160 CDC patients were present in the SEER database from 2001 to 2005. Compared to patients with clear RCC, CDC occurs more frequently in African Americans (23% vs. 9%) [10].

7.4 Clinical Symptoms

Similar to RCC, patients with CDC usually present with abdominal pain, palpable flank mass and gross haematuria. Systemic features as anorexia, weight loss, fatigue and fever are also occasionally present [17]. Approximately one third of patients have metastases at presentation [7]. The most common metastatic sites are the regional lymph nodes, lungs, bone and liver [14].

7.5 Imaging Examinations

Early detection is probably the only factor leading to a prolonged survival for patients with CDC. However, it remains challenging to reliably suggest the diagnosis of CDC based on imaging findings. To date, the imaging features of CDC are not well described, since only case reports or studies involving small numbers of patients have been published [19].

Pickhardt et al. (2001) analysed the radiological observations of 17 patients with histopathologically confirmed CDC. Medullary involvement in small tumours and infiltrative appearance in larger tumours were common findings and may suggest the diagnosis of CDC. In larger tumours, however, these features are frequently associated with an exophytic or expansile component that cannot be distinguished from conventional RCC [20]. Yoon et al. (2006) retrospectively reviewed the CT scans of 18 patients with pathologically proven CDC. The authors reported that medullary location (94%), mild (69%) and heterogeneous (85%) enhancement, involvement of the renal sinus (94%), infiltrative growth (67%), preserved renal contour (61%) and a cystic component (50%) were CT findings frequently observed in CDC patients [21]. More recently, Hu et al. (2014) analysed the imaging features of six CDC patients. The results of the study indicated medullary location, moderate and heterogeneous enhancement, infiltrative growth, damage of renal function in the involved kidney and a marked uptake of ^{18}F-FDG on PET/CT imaging were imaging observations commonly identified. The hypovascular parts of bulky tumours are more likely to be explained by a desmoplastic stromal reaction rather than by tumour necrosis. Nevertheless, these CT findings are non-specific and may not allow CDC to be easily differentiated from other subtypes of RCC. However, when a renal tumour shows these imaging features, CDC may be suggested as a possible differential diagnosis [22]. Figure 7.1 presents contrast enhanced CT images, axial scan and coronal reformatted image, showing a CDC in the upper pole of the left kidney, with lymph node metastasis and pulmonary metastasis.

Also magnetic resonance imaging (MRI) findings are non-specific for CDC. Zhu et al. (2013) retrospectively studied 20 patients with CDC using multisection computed tomography (MSCT) ($n = 20$) or MSCT and MRI ($n = 5$). MRI revealed cystic components, poorly defined tumour borders, isointense tumour on T1-weighted imaging and iso- or hypointense tumour on T2-weighted imaging. Enhancement was reduced within the tumour compared to the renal cortex and medulla [23]. Table 7.1 summarizes the CT and MRI findings frequently observed in CDC patients.

As CDC does not have specific imaging features that distinguish it from other types of RCC, histopathological and immunohistochemical examinations are required for a final diagnosis of CDC.

7.6   Macroscopic Findings

CDCs are usually centrally located within the kidney. When the tumour is small, origin within the renal medulla may be seen. When it is large, irregular extensions into the adjacent renal cortex may be present. Some tumours may extend into the renal pelvis. Local invasion into perirenal and sinus fat can be found. Reported tumour size ranges from 2.5 to 12 cm in diameter (mean 5 cm diameter). They have a grey-white appearance with irregular borders and a firm consistency on sectioning. Tumour necrosis and satellite nodules may be present. Haemorrhage is not usually seen macroscopically [17, 24].

Fig. 7.1 Collecting (Bellini) duct carcinoma: Contrast-enhanced CT images, axial scan (**a**) and coronal reformatted image (**b**) showing a hypovascular infiltrating tumour in the upper pole of the left kidney, with preservation of the renal shape. Metastatic para-aortic lymph nodes (**a**). A lung metastasis is visible at the right diaphragmatic dome (**b**)

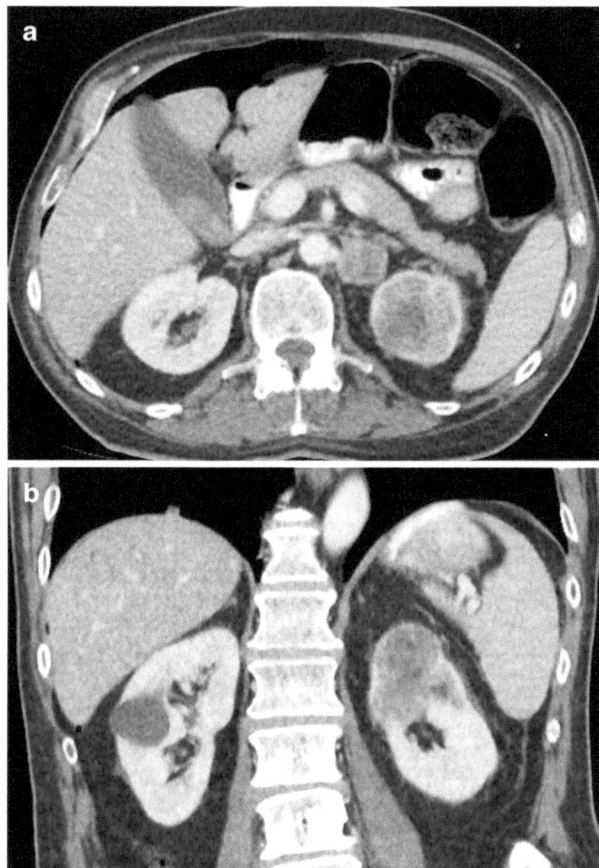

Table 7.1 CT and MRI findings frequently observed in CDC patients

CT	Medullary location
	Mild and heterogenous enhancement
	Involvement of the renal sinus
	Infiltrative growth
	Preserved renal contour
	Cystic component
MSCT or MSCT and MRI	Cystic components
	Poorly defined tumour borders
	Isointense tumour on T1-weighted imaging
	Iso- or hypointense tumour on T2-weighted imaging
	Enhancement reduced within tumour compared to the renal cortex and medulla

CT computed tomography, *MRI* magnetic resonance imaging, *MSCT* multisection computed tomography

7.7   Histopathology

CDC originates from the collecting duct epithelium that arises from the mesoneph-ros (Wolffian duct) as do the ureter, renal pelvis and calyces. It is an ill-defined tumour, consisting of anastomosing tubules, cords and nests of tumour cells, fre-quently with a variety of growth patterns within the same tumour. When extending into the renal cortex, CDC typically infiltrates between the glomeruli, a feature also seen in urothelial cell carcinoma (UCC) but rarely in RCC. Malignant cells have variable amounts of cytoplasm and often pleomorphic nuclei. A 'hobnail' pattern can be present, when the nuclei are apically located within the cells protruding towards the lumen of the tubules. If present, this is a useful characteristic as it is rarely found in other types of RCC (except for type 2 papillary RCC) and not in UCC. Mitotic figures are frequently present. Sarcomatoid dedifferentiation has been reported. Intraluminal mucin production (absent in RCC) staining, positive on peri-odic acid-Schiff (PAS) and mucicarmine stains, can be seen [17]. Atypical cells can be found in adjacent non-invasive distal tubules or collecting ducts, giving a clue to the collecting duct origin of the tumour. The epithelial structures are lying in an abundant, loose or desmoplastic stroma.

In some reported cases, a papillary architecture predominates, giving rise to a differential diagnostic problem with papillary RCC [17]. The clinical and pathobio-logical aspects of CDC and papillary RCC were described in more detail by Kuroda et al. (2002, 2003) [24, 25]. Other differential diagnoses are UCC with glandular differentiation, adenocarcinoma arising from the pelvic urothelium and metastatic carcinoma. As the microscopic appearance of CDC is inconsistent, diagnosis on histological criteria alone is not pathognomonic, and immunohistochemical stain-ing is necessary to show the origin of the tumour [7, 17, 24] (Fig. 7.2).

7.8   Immunohistochemical Findings

CDCs express pankeratin, high molecular weight keratins (HMWK) [34βE12, kera-tin 19 (K19)] and *Ulex europaeus* lectin, as do non-malignant collecting ducts. Tumours usually also show positivity for E-cadherin. Keratin 7 (K7) and epithelial membrane antigen (EMA) reactivity is variable. CD15 (LeuM1), a marker of the proximal tubular epithelium, is negative [7, 14, 17, 26–30]. Other markers of proxi-mal renal tubules (CD10, RCC antigen and α-methylacyl-CoA racemase (AMACR)) are almost always negative [29].

The differential diagnosis of CDC from UCC and papillary RCC is often chal-lenging. The hypothesized association between CDC and UCC, based on similar embryologic origin (mesonephros), has been confirmed in immunohistochemical studies in which both tumour types expressed *Ulex europaeus* lectin and HMWK (both negative in RCC). The three kidney tumours of which two were classified as CDC and one as UCC were negative for cytokeratin 20 (K20) and vimentin [28].

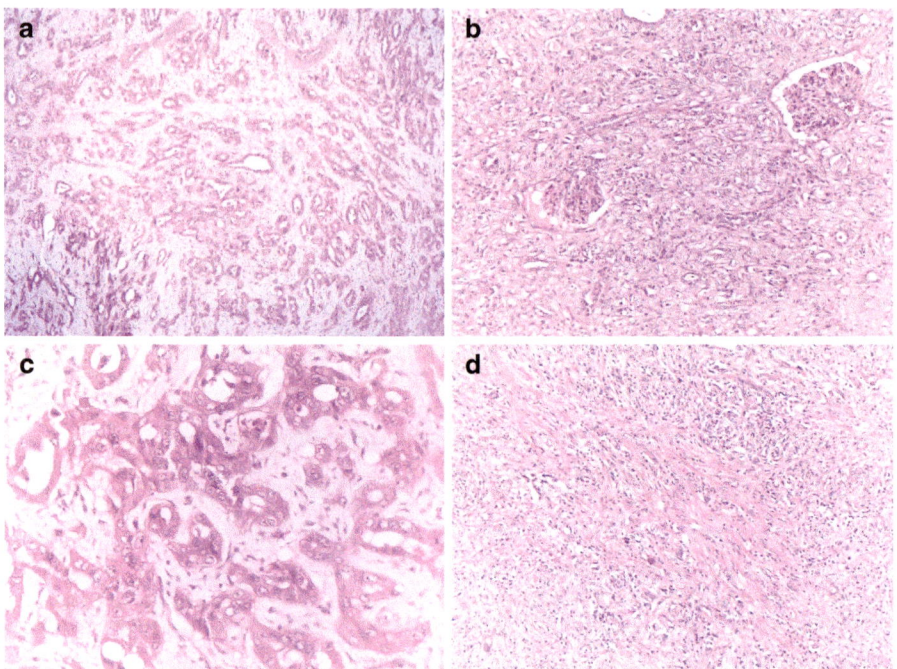

Fig. 7.2 The most typical growth pattern of CDC is a tumour consisting of tubuloglandular structures (panel **a**). However, often the tumour loses this pattern and grows very infiltrative as nests, strands and single cells. This explains the ill-defined borders of CDC. When expanding into the cortex, tumoural cells intersperse between glomeruli (panel **b**). Note the marked nuclear pleomorphism (panel **c**) and the desmoplastic stroma reaction (panel **d**)

Kobayashi et al. (2008) examined the use of adopting immunohistochemical markers for the differential diagnosis of 17 cases of CDC, 10 cases of invasive UCC and 15 cases of papillary RCC. The authors reported that *Ulex europaeus* agglutinin 1 reactivity and positivity for E-cadherin and c-KIT are useful in differentiating CDC from papillary RCC as well as negative results for AMACR and CD10 are potentially useful hallmarks of this distinction. In contrast, using immunohistochemistry with these antigens is not of value in distinguishing CDC and invasive UCC. Therefore, the authors concluded that the differential diagnosis for CDC and invasive UCC requires careful evaluation of clinical information, and macroscopic and microscopic findings, including the intraepithelial lesion of the pelvic urothelial mucosa [31]. Later, Albadine et al. (2010) evaluated the use of the combination of PAX8 and p63 in the differential diagnosis of 21 cases of CDC and 34 cases of upper urinary tract urothelial cell carcinoma (UUT-UCC). The authors showed that the immunoprofile of PAX8+/p63- strongly favoured a diagnosis of CDC, whereas a profile of PAX8−/p63+ favoured UUT-UCC [32]. Gonzalez-Roibon et al. (2013) investigated whether adding the GATA binding protein 3 (GATA3) to this combination might improve its performance in the differential diagnosis of 18 CDC cases and 25 UUT-UCC cases. They found that GATA3 positivity was higher in

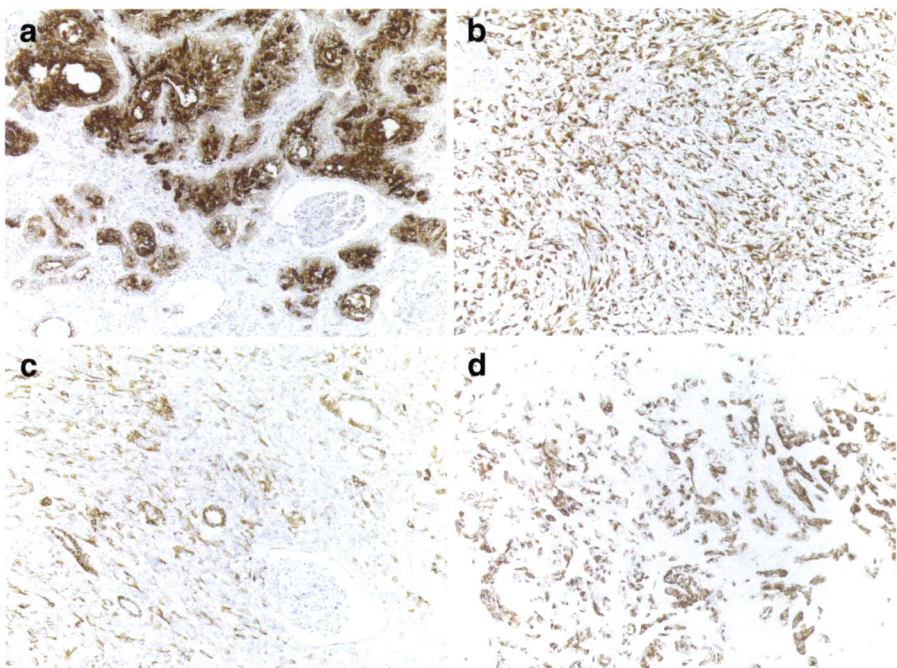

Fig. 7.3 CDC shows cytoplasmic positivity for *Ulex europaeus* lectin (variable staining intensity) (panel **a**). K19 positivity of CDC. In the given case, the picture was taken in an area of pseudosarcomatous dedifferentiation (panel **b**). K7 expression is variable in presence and in staining intensity within CDC (panel **c**). Epithelial membrane antigen (EMA) expression in CDC has been reported as variable. In our hands, it is always positive in CDC (panel **d**)

UUT-UCC (88%) compared to CDC (11%) and that a profile of GATA3 or p63+ and PAX8- strongly favoured a diagnosis of UUT-UCC [33] (Fig. 7.3).

7.9 Diagnostic Criteria

According to the 2016 WHO classification, the diagnostic criteria for CDC are (1) medullary involvement by the tumour, (2) a predominant tubular tumour architecture, (3) epithelial tumoural cells lying within a desmoplastic stroma, (4) high-grade cytology, (5) infiltrative growth pattern and (6) the absence of other renal cell carcinoma subtypes or UCC [9].

7.10 Cytogenetics and Molecular Features

Ancillary cytogenetic techniques, such as conventional karyotyping and fluorescence in situ hybridization (FISH), are not typically helpful for confirmation of diagnosis of CDC. Initial cytogenetic reports are rather confusing, as some have demonstrated mainly a combination of multiple chromosome losses (chromosomes 1, 4, 6, 14, 15, 18 and 20) [34–38], while others described also trisomies and structural chromosomal abnormalities [39, 40]. Cytogenetic biomarkers have not significantly improved the stratification of patients beyond traditional clinical pathologic variables.

More currently, comparative genomic hybridization (CGH) was used to investigate the genetic composition of patient's tumours. In a multicentre German study, Becker et al. (2013) determined genomic copy number alterations of CDC (29 samples) in comparison to those of UUT-UCC (26 samples). The authors showed that CDC was characterized by a different genomic profile compared to UUT-UCC. Recurrent losses of chromosome regions were detected on chromosomes 8p ($n = 9/29$), 16p ($n = 9/29$), 1p ($n = 7/29$) and 9p ($n = 7/29$), and recurrent gains were observed at 13q ($n = 9/29$). Genetic losses on chromosomes 1p36, 3p, 6p and 8p, as well as a gain on chromosome 13, were associated with aggressive disease stages. In contrast to CDC, the most frequently detected UUT-UCC DNA aberration was 9q loss ($n = 13/26$). DNA losses at 13q and 8q as well as gains at 8p showed significant variations in UUT-UCC compared to CDC [41]. The cytogenetic profile of UUT-UCC has been reported to be identical to that of bladder UCC [42, 43]. In addition, CDC is characterized by a different genetic profile compared to three classic RCC histologies, i.e. conventional, papillary and chromophobe RCC [44, 45]. Cytogenetic alterations of RCC and its different subgroups are well documented and generally accepted in many studies published in the last years [46–49]. The study by Becker et al. (2013) suggests CDC as a unique entity among kidney cancers. However, multi-institutional studies of CDC using a larger number of patients are needed to confirm these preliminary findings [41].

Next-generation massively parallel sequencing studies of CDC aimed at understanding the critical molecular alterations associated with this tumour type have been limited due to the tumour rarity. In a recent report, targeted interrogation of genes known to be implicated in cancer was performed in 17 locally advanced or metastatic CDC tumours. Thirty-six genomic alterations were detected, the most common being *NF2*/22q12 (29%), *SETD2*/3p21.1 (24%), *SMARCB1*/22q11 (18%) and *CDKN2A*/9p21 (12%). In addition, mutations of *PIK3CA*, *PIK3R2*, *FBXW7*, *BAP1*, *DNMT3A*, *VHL* and *HRAS* were also identified in single cases. Notably, these mutations were defined as clinically relevant given their ability to aid in selection of approved targeted therapies [50]. Recent whole exome sequencing and RNA-seq analysis of 7 CDC tumours, as well as additional FISH analysis of *CDKN2A* on 16 tumours, confirmed the frequent loss of *CDKN2A* (62.5% of cases) [51]. Understanding the molecular pathogenesis of CDC will play a key role in the future subclassification of this unique tumour.

7.11 Treatment

Multi-institutional collaboration is required to assemble a sufficiently large number of cases to make statements on possible treatments. Three studies [14–16] relevant to the management of CDC were identified in a systematic review by Dason et al. [52].

7.11.1 Surgery

Evidence for the role of surgery is lacking in the literature. Almost all reported patients with CDC underwent surgery [10, 12, 14, 15, 53] and were diagnosed with CDC after histopathology examination [10, 14, 15, 53]. Eighty-seven percent of the patients in the study of Oudard et al. underwent prior cytoreductive nephrectomy [15]. Mejean et al. (2003) reported three perioperative deaths in their series of ten patients undergoing surgery for CDC. They concluded that because the prognosis is poor despite radical nephrectomy, biopsy should be performed first when radiological findings are suggestive of CDC. For metastatic CDC (mCDC), radical nephrectomy alone does not seem to be useful except for palliative reasons or in combination with new chemotherapy regimen [54]. Abern et al. (2012) examined 227 CDC cases and reported that CDC patients selected for cytoreductive nephrectomy had improved survival [11]. As most CDC patients are already metastatic at presentation, the rate of perioperative morbidity is high and may delay or prevent the patients from receiving systemic treatment [15]. Accordingly, surgical therapy for CDC must be individualized.

7.11.2 Chemotherapy

Based on the clinical similarities between CDC and UCC, Milowsky et al. (2002) suggested that the chemotherapy regimen used for treatment of UCC might also be appropriate for CDC [55]. A prospective multicentre phase II study with central histopathology review evaluated the effect of gemcitabine and either cisplatin or carboplatin (GC) on 23 patients with mCDC. The objective response rate was 26% (95% CI 8–44). Median progression-free survival (PFS) and overall survival (OS) were 7.1 (95% CI 3–11.3) and 10.5 months (95% CI 3.8–17.1), respectively. Of the 23 patients, 87% underwent cytoreductive nephrectomy, and 96% had Eastern Cooperative Oncology Group (ECOG) performance status ≤ 2 [15]. It is unknown how the study results would have been in patients who did not undergo surgery. The treatment was associated with manageable adverse events. Toxicity was mainly haematological with grade 3–4 neutropenia and thrombocytopenia in 52% and 43% of patients, respectively. Given the lack of any other beneficial agent, this platinum-based chemotherapy regimen should be considered the standard of care for first-line systemic treatment of mCDC patients [15].

In 2012, a case report presented complete remission of pulmonary metastases and long-term survival in a mCDC patient treated with gemcitabine, cisplatin and bevacizumab [56]. In a more recent study, five patients diagnosed with mCDC received bevacizumab in addition of the GC combination. All patients had undergone radical nephrectomy, but none had received previous systemic treatment for CDC. This new triple treatment regimen resulted in a longer PFS (15.1 months, 95% CI 5.6–20.4) and longer OS (27.8 months, 95% CI 12.4–unreached) (more than double) than recorded in 2007 by Oudard et al. in patients treated with a GC regimen. The French Collaborative Group is currently recruiting patients in a prospective multicentre phase II study (NCT02363751) of this triple treatment regimen in mCDC [57]. Case reports have also reported responses to paclitaxel [58] and paclitaxel and carboplatin [59].

7.11.3 Immunotherapy

The largest series of CDC treated with immunotherapy is a retrospective series based on a multi-institutional survey (66 Japanese centres) that comprised 81 patients and was confirmed by a central review. In a subpopulation of this study, immunotherapy was used in 34 CDC patients (interferon (IFN-α, INF-γ) or interleukin 2 (IL-2)). No responses were observed [14]. Also in another retrospective study including 15 CDC patients treated with immunotherapy, no therapy effect was recorded [16]. The programmed death-1 and programmed death-ligand 1 (PD-1/PD-L1) targeting antibodies, alone or in combination with anti-angiogenic drugs or other immunotherapeutic approaches, show promising results for the treatment of RCC. A recent study suggested that PD-L1 could represent an important therapeutic target for CDC. However, only 5 of the 101 non-clear cell RCCs in this study were CDC. One of five CDCs were considered PD-L1+, and PD-L1 positivity by tumour-infiltrating mononuclear cells was observed in all 5 CDCs [60]. The efficacy and safety of anti-PD-1/PD-L1 agents in specific RCC subpopulations such as CDC patients should be further investigated [61].

7.11.4 Targeted Therapy

Staehler et al. (2008) reported no response to sunitinib in two patients with mCDC [62]. Miyake et al. (2011) presented a case report of partial response of mCDC after sunitinib therapy [63]. Procopio et al. (2012) reported a series of seven patients receiving targeted therapies (sorafenib, temsirolimus and sunitinib). Two patients experienced a period of disease stabilization with an overall survival time of 49 (sorafenib followed by sunitinib) and 19 months (temsirolimus followed by sunitinib), respectively [64]. Two case reports showed response of mCDC after sorafenib therapy [65, 66].

There is no evidence to support the efficacy of targeted therapy, such as sunitinib and sorafenib beyond small series. Prospectively investigating the role of targeted therapy in the management of mCDC would be valuable.

Table 7.2 summarizes the main studies of therapeutic regimens for CDC.

7.12   Prognosis and Predictive Factors

Three multi-institutional retrospective studies were published from the United States [10], Europe [12] and Japan [14] showing that CDC presents usually at an advanced stage and has a poor prognosis, due to the frequent finding of distant metastases at the time of diagnosis [7, 10, 13, 14, 17, 26–28, 53, 67–72].

Table 7.2 Summary of the main studies of therapeutic regimens for CDC

References	Therapeutic regimen	Outcome
Tokuda et al. [14]	Immunotherapy Chemotherapy	No responses 1 PR to gemcitabine/carboplatin 1-, 3-, 5- and 10-year disease-specific survival 69.0%, 45.3%, 34.3% and 13.7%
Oudard et al. [15]	Gemcitabine/platinum	Objective response rate 26% (95% CI 8–44) 1 CR, 5 PR, 10 SD and 7 PD Median OS: 10.5 mo (95% CI 3.8–17.1) Median PFS: 7.1 mo (95% CI 3.0–11.3)
Procopio et al. [64]	4 patients on sorafenib 1 patient on sunitinib 2 patients on temsirolimus	Long-lasting disease control 1 patient had OS of 49 mo (sorafenib followed by sunitinib) 1 patient had OS of 19 mo (temsirolimus followed by sunitinib)
Pécuchet et al. [57]	Bevacizumab + gemcitabine + platinum salt	3 PR and 2 SD Median OS: 27.8 mo (95% CI 12.4–unreached) Median PFS: 15.1 mo (95% CI 5.6–20.4)

CR complete response, *PR* partial response, *SD* stable disease, *PD* progressive disease, *OS* overall survival, *PFS* progression-free survival, *mo* months

Early diagnosis is therefore important and may increase survival. A high frequency of local recurrence is reported, even when a radical nephrectomy has been successfully performed [24].

In the Japanese study, with a series of 81 CDC patients, regional lymph node metastases were detected in 44% of the patients, while 32% of the population had distant metastases at presentation. The 5-year disease-specific survival was 34.3% [14].

In the European multi-institutional surgical series, CDC patients presented with more advanced stage and more aggressive disease compared to clear cell RCC patients. Of all CDC patients, 76% had pT3 disease at nephrectomy versus 37% for those with clear cell RCC. The predominant Fuhrman grades were III (56%) and IV (22%) in CDC patients versus II (42%) and III (28%) for clear cell RCC patients. Of all CDC patients, 19% had distant metastases at nephrectomy compared to 14% of the clear cell RCC patients. After nephrectomy, when 41 CDC cases were matched for grade, tumour size and TNM stages with 105 clear cell RCC controls, no difference in 5-year disease-specific survival was observed (48% and 57%, respectively). An explanation for this paradox cannot be offered readily and may require more information on the tumour biology of CDC [12].

On analysis of the Surveillance, Epidemiology, and End Results (SEER) database for the years 2001–2005, i.e. before the introduction of anti-angiogenic drugs, mortality for CDC (n = 160) was 2.42-fold higher than for clear cell RCC (n = 33,252). The 3-year disease-specific survival rate was 58% and 79% for CDC and clear cell RCC, respectively [10].

In the study by Oudard et al. including 23 patients with mCDC on a GC regimen, 66% of patients died of the disease within 2 years after diagnosis [15]. Recently, a multi-institutional study with 95 CDC patients collected from 16 European and American centres reported a 5-year disease-specific survival of 40.3% with a median follow-up time of 48.1 months. The authors assessed the parameters prognostic for disease-specific mortality: American Society of Anesthesiologists (ASA) score 3–4, tumour size greater than 7 cm, stage M1, Fuhrman grade 3–4 and lymphovascular invasion. Based on these parameters, patients were divided into 26 (27%) at low-risk (0–2 points), 13 (14%) at intermediate-risk (3 points) and 56 patients (59%) at high-risk group (4–7 points) with a 5-year disease-specific survival of 96%, 62% and 8%, respectively ($P < 0.001$). A subset of low-risk patients has excellent survival when histopathological parameters in a highly accurate risk model were used to stratify the patients [13]. A recent multi-institutional study that examined the treatment results in 35 CDC patients showed seven long-term survivors. Long-term survivors were in stages I–III and those who received palliative treatment after a relapse. The treatments administered to these patients included targeted therapy as well as immunotherapy and chemotherapy. Therefore, additional research on predictive markers, by which the outcomes of prognosis and therapy as well as their clinical features can be predicted, is needed [53].

Conclusion

CDC is a rare and aggressive subtype of RCC arising from the principal cells of the collecting duct epithelium. It presents at an advanced stage and has an extremely poor prognosis. Imaging features of CDC are non-specific.

Light microscopy findings are typically described as a cytologically high grade, tubular or tubulopapillary growing carcinoma within a desmoplastic stroma. Histological and immunohistochemical analyses, together with clinical data, are critical in establishing an accurate diagnosis of CDC and for distinguishing this tumour from other subtypes of RCC.

Understanding the molecular pathogenesis of CDC will play a key role in the future subclassification of this unique tumour. Most of the CDC patients receive surgical treatment although evidence for the role of surgery is lacking in the literature. Several other treatments including chemotherapy, radiotherapy and immunotherapy have been considered but have a poor response. Given the lack of any other beneficial agent, a GC regimen should be considered the standard of care for first-line systemic treatment of mCDC patients. The role of targeted therapy in the management of CDC has not been established because of the limited data to date.

Early diagnosis, additional research on predictive markers and prospective multi-institutional studies to investigate treatments of CDC will be necessary to improve the outcome of these patients.

References

1. Storkel S, Eble JN, Adlakha K, Amin M, Blute ML, Bostwick DG, et al. Classification of renal cell carcinoma: workgroup No. 1. Union Internationale Contre le Cancer (UICC) and the American Joint Committee on Cancer (AJCC). Cancer. 1997;80(5):987–9.
2. Polascik TJ, Cairns P, Epstein JI, Fuzesi L, Ro JY, Marshall FF, et al. Distal nephron renal tumors: microsatellite allelotype. Cancer Res. 1996;56(8):1892–5.
3. Mancilla-Jimenez R, Stanley RJ, Blath RA. Papillary renal cell carcinoma: a clinical, radiologic, and pathologic study of 34 cases. Cancer. 1976;38(6):2469–80.
4. Thoenes W, Storkel S, Rumpelt HJ. Histopathology and classification of renal cell tumors (adenomas, oncocytomas and carcinomas). The basic cytological and histopathological elements and their use for diagnostics. Pathol Res Pract. 1986;181(2):125–43.
5. Fleming S, Lewi HJ. Collecting duct carcinoma of the kidney. Histopathology. 1986;10(11):1131–41.
6. Kovacs G, Akhtar M, Beckwith BJ, Bugert P, Cooper CS, Delahunt B, et al. The Heidelberg classification of renal cell tumours. J Pathol. 1997;183(2):131–3.
7. Eble JN, Sauter G, Epstein JI, Sesterhenn IA, editors. Tumours of the urinary and male genital organs. Lyon: IARC; 2004.
8. Cornelis F, Helenon O, Correas JM, Lemaitre L, Andre M, Meuwly JY, et al. Tubulocystic renal cell carcinoma: a new radiological entity. Eur Radiol. 2016;26(4):1108–15.
9. Moch H, Cubilla AL, Humphrey PA, Reuter VE, Ulbright TM. The 2016 WHO classification of Tumours of the urinary system and male genital organs-part a: renal, penile, and testicular tumours. Eur Urol. 2016;70(1):93–105.
10. Wright JL, Risk MC, Hotaling J, Lin DW. Effect of collecting duct histology on renal cell cancer outcome. J Urol. 2009;182(6):2595–9.
11. Abern MR, Tsivian M, Polascik TJ, Coogan CL. Characteristics and outcomes of tumors arising from the distal nephron. Urology. 2012;80(1):140–6.
12. Karakiewicz PI, Trinh QD, Rioux-Leclercq N, de la Taille A, Novara G, Tostain J, et al. Collecting duct renal cell carcinoma: a matched analysis of 41 cases. Eur Urol. 2007;52(4):1140–5.
13. May M, Ficarra V, Shariat SF, Zigeuner R, Chromecki T, Cindolo L, et al. Impact of clinical and histopathological parameters on disease specific survival in patients with collecting duct renal cell carcinoma: development of a disease specific risk model. J Urol. 2013;190(2):458–63.
14. Tokuda N, Naito S, Matsuzaki O, Nagashima Y, Ozono S, Igarashi T. Collecting duct (Bellini duct) renal cell carcinoma: a nationwide survey in Japan. J Urol. 2006;176(1):40–3. discussion 3
15. Oudard S, Banu E, Vieillefond A, Fournier L, Priou F, Medioni J, et al. Prospective multicenter phase II study of gemcitabine plus platinum salt for metastatic collecting duct carcinoma: results of a GETUG (Groupe d'Etudes des Tumeurs Uro-Genitales) study. J Urol. 2007;177(5):1698–702.
16. Motzer RJ, Bacik J, Mariani T, Russo P, Mazumdar M, Reuter V. Treatment outcome and survival associated with metastatic renal cell carcinoma of non-clear-cell histology. J Clin Oncol. 2002;20(9):2376–81.
17. Srigley JR, Eble JN. Collecting duct carcinoma of kidney. Semin Diagn Pathol. 1998;15(1):54–67.
18. Pepek JM, Johnstone PA, Jani AB. Influence of demographic factors on outcome of collecting duct carcinoma: a surveillance, epidemiology, and end results (SEER) database analysis. Clin Genitourin Cancer. 2009;7(2):E24–7.
19. Oyen R, Verswijvel G, Van Poppel H, Roskams T. Primary malignant renal parenchymal epithelial neoplasms. Radiologic-pathologic correlations. Eur Radiol. 2000;10(Suppl 2):S 231–43.

20. Pickhardt PJ, Siegel CL, McLarney JK. Collecting duct carcinoma of the kidney: are imaging findings suggestive of the diagnosis? AJR Am J Roentgenol. 2001;176(3):627–33.
21. Yoon SK, Nam KJ, Rha SH, Kim JK, Cho KS, Kim B, et al. Collecting duct carcinoma of the kidney: CT and pathologic correlation. Eur J Radiol. 2006;57(3):453–60.
22. Hu Y, Lu GM, Li K, Zhang LJ, Zhu H. Collecting duct carcinoma of the kidney: imaging observations of a rare tumor. Oncol Lett. 2014;7(2):519–24.
23. Zhu Q, Wu J, Wang Z, Zhu W, Chen W, Wang S. The MSCT and MRI findings of collecting duct carcinoma. Clin Radiol. 2013;68(10):1002–7.
24. Kuroda N, Toi M, Hiroi M, Enzan H. Review of collecting duct carcinoma with focus on clinical and pathobiological aspects. Histol Histopathol. 2002;17(4):1329–34.
25. Kuroda N, Toi M, Hiroi M, Enzan H. Review of papillary renal cell carcinoma with focus on clinical and pathobiological aspects. Histol Histopathol. 2003;18(2):487–94.
26. Matei DV, Rocco B, Varela R, Verweij F, Scardino E, Renne G, et al. Synchronous collecting duct carcinoma and papillary renal cell carcinoma: a case report and review of the literature. Anticancer Res. 2005;25(1B):579–86.
27. Dobronski P, Czaplicki M, Kozminska E, Pykalo R. Collecting (Bellini) duct carcinoma of the kidney—clinical, radiologic and immunohistochemical findings. Int Urol Nephrol. 1999;31(5):601–9.
28. Orsola A, Trias I, Raventos CX, Espanol I, Cecchini L, Orsola I. Renal collecting (Bellini) duct carcinoma displays similar characteristics to upper tract urothelial cell carcinoma. Urology. 2005;65(1):49–54.
29. Srigley JR, Delahunt B. Uncommon and recently described renal carcinomas. Mod Pathol. 2009;22(Suppl 2):S2–S23.
30. Oyen R, Verswijvel G, Van Poppel H, Roskams T. Primary malignant renal parenchymal epithelial neoplasms. Eur Radiol. 2001;11(Suppl 2):S205–S17.
31. Kobayashi N, Matsuzaki O, Shirai S, Aoki I, Yao M, Nagashima Y. Collecting duct carcinoma of the kidney: an immunohistochemical evaluation of the use of antibodies for differential diagnosis. Hum Pathol. 2008;39(9):1350–9.
32. Albadine R, Schultz L, Illei P, Ertoy D, Hicks J, Sharma R, et al. PAX8 (+)/p63 (−) immunostaining pattern in renal collecting duct carcinoma (CDC): a useful immunoprofile in the differential diagnosis of CDC versus urothelial carcinoma of upper urinary tract. Am J Surg Pathol. 2010;34(7):965–9.
33. Gonzalez-Roibon N, Albadine R, Sharma R, Faraj SF, Illei PB, Argani P, et al. The role of GATA binding protein 3 in the differential diagnosis of collecting duct and upper tract urothelial carcinomas. Hum Pathol. 2013;44(12):2651–7.
34. Füzesi L, Cober M, Mittermayer C. Collecting duct carcinoma: cytogenetic characterization. Histopathology. 1992;21(2):155–60.
35. Schoenberg M, Cairns P, Brooks JD, Marshall FF, Epstein JI, Isaacs WB, et al. Frequent loss of chromosome arms 8p and 13q in collecting duct carcinoma (CDC) of the kidney. Genes Chromosomes Cancer. 1995;12(1):76–80.
36. Verdorfer I, Culig Z, Hobisch A, Bartsch G, Hittmair A, Duba HC, et al. Characterisation of a collecting duct carcinoma by cytogenetic analysis and comparative genomic hybridisation. Int J Oncol. 1998;13(3):461–4.
37. Antonelli A, Portesi E, Cozzoli A, Zanotelli T, Tardanico R, Balzarini P, et al. The collecting duct carcinoma of the kidney: a cytogenetical study. Eur Urol. 2003;43(6):680–5.
38. Parker R, Reeves HM, Sudarshan S, Wolff D, Keane T. Abnormal fluorescence in situ hybridization analysis in collecting duct carcinoma. Urology. 2005;66(5):1110.
39. Cavazzana AO, Prayer-Galetti T, Tirabosco R, Macciomei MC, Stella M, Lania L, et al. Bellini duct carcinoma. A clinical and in vitro study. Eur Urol. 1996;30(3):340–4.
40. Gregon-Romero MA, Morell-Quadreny L, Llombart-Bosch A. Cytogenetic analysis of three primary Bellini duct carcinoma. Genes Chromosomes Cancer. 1996;15:170–2.
41. Becker F, Junker K, Parr M, Hartmann A, Fussel S, Toma M, et al. Collecting duct carcinomas represent a unique tumor entity based on genetic alterations. PLoS One. 2013;8(10):e78137.

42. Marin-Aguilera M, Mengual L, Ribal MJ, Musquera M, Ars E, Villavicencio H, et al. Utility of fluorescence in situ hybridization as a non-invasive technique in the diagnosis of upper urinary tract urothelial carcinoma. Eur Urol. 2007;51(2):409–15. discussion 15

43. Fadl-Elmula I, Gorunova L, Mandahl N, Elfving P, Lundgren R, Rademark C, et al. Cytogenetic analysis of upper urinary tract transitional cell carcinomas. Cancer Genet Cytogenet. 1999;115(2):123–7.

44. Junker K, Weirich G, Amin MB, Moravek P, Hindermann W, Schubert J. Genetic subtyping of renal cell carcinoma by comparative genomic hybridization. Recent Results Cancer Res. 2003;162:169–75.

45. Wilhelm M, Veltman JA, Olshen AB, Jain AN, Moore DH, Presti JC Jr, et al. Array-based comparative genomic hybridization for the differential diagnosis of renal cell cancer. Cancer Res. 2002;62(4):957–60.

46. Meloni-Ehrig AM. Renal cancer: cytogenetic and molecular genetic aspects. Am J Med Genet. 2002;115(3):164–72.

47. Dondeti VR, Wubbenhorst B, Lal P, Gordan JD, D'Andrea K, Attiyeh EF, et al. Integrative genomic analyses of sporadic clear cell renal cell carcinoma define disease subtypes and potential new therapeutic targets. Cancer Res. 2012;72(1):112–21.

48. Girgis AH, Iakovlev VV, Beheshti B, Bayani J, Squire JA, Bui A, et al. Multilevel whole-genome analysis reveals candidate biomarkers in clear cell renal cell carcinoma. Cancer Res. 2012;72(20):5273–84.

49. Pei J, Feder MM, Al-Saleem T, Liu Z, Liu A, Hudes GR, et al. Combined classical cytogenetics and microarray-based genomic copy number analysis reveal frequent 3;5 rearrangements in clear cell renal cell carcinoma. Genes Chromosomes Cancer. 2010;49(7):610–9.

50. Pal SK, Choueiri TK, Wang K, Khaira D, Karam JA, Van Allen E, et al. Characterization of clinical cases of collecting duct carcinoma of the kidney assessed by comprehensive genomic profiling. Eur Urol. 2016;70(3):516–21.

51. Wang JZ, Papanicolau-Sengos A, Chintala S, Wei L, Liu B, Hu Q. Collecting duct carcinoma of the kidney is associated with CDKN2A deletion and SLC family gene up-regulation. Oncotarget. 2016;7(21):29901–15. https://doi.org/10.18632/oncotarget.9093.

52. Dason S, Allard C, Sheridan-Jonah A, Gill J, Jamshaid H, Aziz T, Kajal B, Kapoor A. Management of renal collecting duct carcinoma: a systematic review and the McMaster experience. Curr Oncol. 2013;20:223–32.

53. Kwon KA, Oh SY, Kim HY, Kim HS, Lee HY, Kim TM, et al. Clinical features and treatment of collecting duct carcinoma of the kidney from the korean cancer study group genitourinary and gynecology cancer committee. Cancer Res Treat. 2014;46(2):141–7.

54. Mejean A, Roupret M, Larousserie F, Hopirtean V, Thiounn N, Dufour B. Is there a place for radical nephrectomy in the presence of metastatic collecting duct (Bellini) carcinoma? J Urol. 2003;169(4):1287–90.

55. Milowsky MI, Rosmarin A, Tickoo SK, Papanicolaou N, Nanus DM. Active chemotherapy for collecting duct carcinoma of the kidney: a case report and review of the literature. Cancer. 2002;94(1):111–6.

56. Barrascout E, Beuselinck B, Ayllon J, Battig B, Moch H, Teghom C, et al. Complete remission of pulmonary metastases of Bellini duct carcinoma with cisplatin, gemcitabine and bevacizumab. Am J Case Rep. 2012;13:1–2.

57. Pécuchet N, Bigot F, Gachet J, Massard C, Albiges L, Teghom C, et al. Triple combination of bevacizumab, gemcitabine and platinum salt in metastatic collecting duct carcinoma. Ann Oncol. 2013;24(12):2963–7.

58. Bagrodia A, Gold R, Handorf C, Liman A, Derweesh IH. Salvage paclitaxel chemotherapy for metastatic collecting duct carcinoma of the kidney. Can J Urol. 2008;15(6):4425–7.

59. Gollob JA, Upton MP, DeWolf WC, Atkins MB. Long-term remission in a patient with metastatic collecting duct carcinoma treated with taxol/carboplatin and surgery. Urology. 2001;58(6):1058.

60. Choueiri TK, Fay AP, Gray KP, Callea M, Ho TH, Albiges L, et al. PD-L1 expression in nonclear-cell renal cell carcinoma. Ann Oncol. 2014;25(11):2178–84.

61. Massari F, Santoni M, Ciccarese C, Santini D, Alfieri S, Martignoni G, et al. PD-1 blockade therapy in renal cell carcinoma: current studies and future promises. Cancer Treat Rev. 2015;41(2):114–21.
62. Staehler M, Haseke N, Schoppler G, Stadler T, Karl A, Siebels M, et al. Carcinoma of the collecting ducts of Bellini of the kidney: adjuvant chemotherapy followed by multikinase-inhibition with sunitinib. Eur J Med Res. 2008;13(11):531–5.
63. Miyake H, Haraguchi T, Takenaka A, Fujisawa M. Metastatic collecting duct carcinoma of the kidney responded to sunitinib. Int J Clin Oncol. 2011;16(2):153–5.
64. Procopio G, Verzoni E, Iacovelli R, Colecchia M, Torelli T, Mariani L. Is there a role for targeted therapies in the collecting ducts of Bellini carcinoma? Efficacy data from a retrospective analysis of 7 cases. Clin Exp Nephrol. 2012;16(3):464–7.
65. Ansari J, Fatima A, Chaudhri S, Bhatt RI, Wallace M, James ND. Sorafenib induces therapeutic response in a patient with metastatic collecting duct carcinoma of kidney. Onkologie. 2009;32(1–2):44–6.
66. Zhao RN, Nie LH, Gong R, Wang JZ, Wazir R, Liu LR, et al. Active targeted therapy for metastatic collecting duct carcinoma of the kidney: a case report and review of the literature. Int Urol Nephrol. 2013;45(4):1017–21.
67. Wang X, Hao J, Zhou R, Zhang X, Yan T, Ding D, et al. Collecting duct carcinoma of the kidney: a clinicopathological study of five cases. Diagn Pathol. 8:96.
68. Chao D, Zisman A, Pantuck AJ, Gitlitz BJ, Freedland SJ, Said JW, et al. Collecting duct renal cell carcinoma: clinical study of a rare tumor. J Urol. 2002;167(1):71–4.
69. Kennedy SM, Merino MJ, Linehan WM, Roberts JR, Robertson CN, Neumann RD. Collecting duct carcinoma of the kidney. Hum Pathol. 1990;21(4):449–56.
70. Rumpelt HJ, Storkel S, Moll R, Scharfe T, Thoenes W. Bellini duct carcinoma: further evidence for this rare variant of renal cell carcinoma. Histopathology. 1991;18(2):115–22.
71. Amin MB, Tamboli P, Javidan J, Stricker H, de-Peralta Venturina M, Deshpande A, et al. Prognostic impact of histologic subtyping of adult renal epithelial neoplasms: an experience of 405 cases. Am J Surg Pathol. 2002;26(3):281–91.
72. Ciszewski S, Jakimow A, Smolska-Ciszewska B. Collecting (Bellini) duct carcinoma: a clinical study of a rare tumour and review of the literature. Can Urol Assoc J. 2015;9(9–10):E589–93.

TFE/Translocation Morphology Renal Cell Carcinoma

8

James I. Geller, Nicholas G. Cost, and Mariana M. Cajaiba

8.1 Introduction

TFE/translocation renal cell carcinoma (tRCC) was formally recognized by the WHO in 2004 as a distinct, typically translocation-associated, RCC with characteristic morphology and immunohistochemical expression of TFE3 or TFEb. Cytogenetic translocations may include TFE3-ASPS, TFE3-PRCC, TFEb-alpha, or other variants; mechanisms for TFE upregulation may be heterogenous. TFE3 and TFEB are members of the MiTF/TFE family of basic helix-loop-helix-leucine zipper transcription factors [1–3].

8.2 Epidemiology and Clinical Presentation

tRCCs tend to present at a younger age but may present at any age. Approximately half of Paediatric RCCs are tRCCs, with a slight female predominance [4–6]. tRCC presents in all races, accounting for 1–5% of RCC overall [4, 7–11].

The dominant presentation pattern of tRCC is one of advanced stage and rapid fatality, pointing to an aggressive cancer [12, 13], though infrequent late recurrences [14] and prolonged stable disease [4, 15, 16] point to a less common indolent pattern. Overall, in Paediatric series, approximately 65% of tRCC cases present with

J. I. Geller (✉)
Cincinnati Children's Hospital Medical Center, University of Cincinnati, Cincinnati, OH, USA
e-mail: James.Geller@cchmc.org

N. G. Cost
Division of Urology, Department of Surgery, Children's Hospital Colorado, University of Colorado Cancer Center, Aurora, CO, USA

M. M. Cajaiba
Department of Pathology, University of Michigan, Ann Arbor, MI, USA

© Springer Nature Switzerland AG 2019
G. G. Malouf, N. M. Tannir (eds.), *Rare Kidney Tumors*,
https://doi.org/10.1007/978-3-319-96989-3_8

TNM Stage 3 or 4 disease [5]. For tRCC adult patient cohorts published by medical oncologists, referral patterns may have an impact on stage distribution since low-stage cases are not often referred by urologic oncologists [9, 10].

The import of frequent positive lymph nodes, with high rates of 41% in younger cohorts [4, 5] and up to 50–80% in older tRCC cohorts [9, 10], is debated, with reports suggesting both a favorable [4, 11, 17] and unfavorable outcome [10]. Nodal disease is also common with small primary tumors, with rates ranging from 20 to 33% for T1/T2 disease [5, 6, 11]. Rates of hematogenous metastatic disease range from 9% [5, 11] to 35–75% in select older tRCC cohorts [10].

8.3   Molecular Biology

tRCCs are characterized by the presence of gene rearrangements involving the *TFE3* (Xp11.2) or *TFEB* (6p21) genes. Both genes are members of the microphthalmia transcription factor (MiT) family, together with *TFEC* (7q31) and *MITF* (3p13). These four genes encode basic helix-loop-helix-leucine zipper transcription factors and share homology of their binding domains resulting in activation of common downstream targets [18]. Among the MiT family genes, *MITF* has been well characterized as a key regulator of melanocyte differentiation [19, 20].

Rearrangements involving *TFE3* and *TFEB* result in fusion of these genes with promoters of partner genes, leading to increased *TFE3* and *TFEB* transcription and upregulation of their binding domains [21, 22]. As a result, oncogenic transformation in tRCC is expected to occur following enhanced activation of downstream targets of *TFE3* and *TFEB* which are involved in cell proliferation and survival [23]. As an example, *TFE3* gene fusion transcripts have been shown to activate the MET tyrosine kinase pathway through upregulation of the *MET* gene [24]. Other target genes activated by members of the MiT family and involved in cell growth and survival include *Bcl2, CDK2, HIF1A*, and *CYCLIN E* [25–28]. Additionally, TFE3 chimeric proteins have also been shown to induce loss of cell cycle control due to downregulation of the Mad2B and p53 proteins [29, 30].

Multiple genes have been identified as *TFE3* fusion partners in TRCC, with *PRCC* (1q21) and *ASPL* (or *ASPSCR1*, 17q25) being the most frequently reported. Of interest, *ASPL-TFE3* fusion transcripts have also been identified in alveolar soft part sarcomas [31]. Less commonly reported partner genes include *CLTC* (17q23), *SFPQ* (or *PSF*, 1p34), *NONO* (or *p54nrb*, Xq12), *PARP14* (3q21), *LUC7L3* (17q21), *KHSRP* (19p13), and *DVL2* (17p13) [32]. In contrast to the numerous fusion partners reported for *TFE3*, all reported cases of tRCC with *TFEB* fusions had the *MALAT1* (or *Alpha*, 11q13) gene as the fusion partner.

Although *TFE3* and *TFEB* gene rearrangements were originally identified through conventional karyotype, they can also be detected in formalin-fixed paraffin-embedded (FFPE) material using interphase fluorescence in situ hybridization (FISH) with telomeric and centromeric (break-apart) probes designed to flank these genes [33, 34]. Split signals for these probes indicate gene rearrangement, in contrast to fused signals in normal cases. RT-PCR assays with primers designed for specific fusion transcripts can also be performed using RNA extracted from FFPE tissue [35, 36]. In addition, RNA next-generation sequencing (NGS) techniques can also detect these gene rearrangements in FFPE tissue, with the advantage of allowing identification of unknown fusion partners [32, 37].

8.4 Pathology

Histologically, tRCC typically shows a characteristic combination of morphological features that helps to distinguish these tumors from other types of RCC. Tumors with *TFE3* fusion transcripts are characterized by a predominance of polygonal cells with abundant clear cytoplasm admixed with variable amounts of cells showing granular eosinophilic cytoplasm (Fig. 8.1a–c). Some tumors show an abrupt transition between areas with clear and eosinophilic cytoplasm, and a predominance of eosinophilic cytoplasm can also occur. Most cases correspond to ISUP nuclear grades 2 and 3. Papillary and nested growth patterns are seen in variable proportions in these neoplasms (Fig. 8.1a, b) and often occur within the same tumor, and

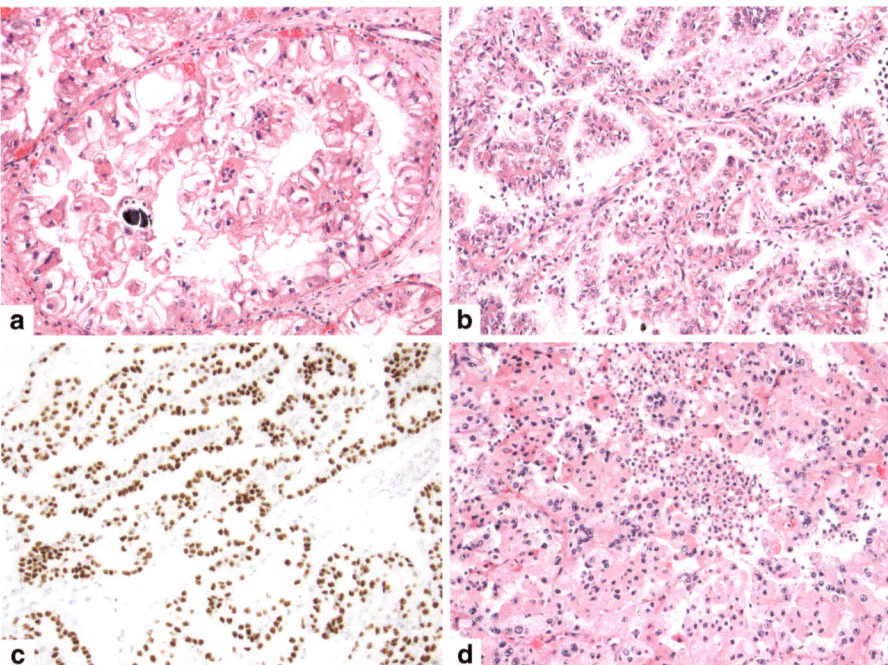

Fig. 8.1 tRCCs with *TFE3* fusion transcripts composed of cells with abundant clear and/or eosinophilic cytoplasm arranged in nested (**a**) and papillary (**b**) growth patterns. Strong nuclear TFE3 immunohistochemical expression in a tRCC bearing a *TFE3* fusion transcript (**c**). Biphasic cell population consisting of large and small cells seen in a tRCC with a *TFEB* fusion transcript (**d**)

compact solid architecture and focal cystic areas can be seen in a small subset of tumors. Psammomatous calcifications are frequently appreciated.

Some morphological features appear to be more frequently associated with specific partner genes involved in the *TFE3* fusion [38]. Larger cells with voluminous cell cytoplasm and well-defined cell membranes reminiscent of "plant" cells, as well as more numerous psammoma bodies, are features more frequently described in cases with the *ASPL-TFE3* fusion transcript. In contrast, cases bearing *PRCC-TFE3* fusion transcripts frequently show smaller cells with less voluminous cytoplasm and indistinct cell membranes. Subnuclear vacuoles and nuclear palisading have been described as distinctive features occurring in cases with *SFPQ-TFE3* and *NONO-TFE3* fusion transcripts [32].

Most tumors with *TFEB* fusion transcripts show a peculiar biphasic cell population characterized by large cells with eosinophilic and granular to clear cytoplasm admixed with less numerous small cells with little cytoplasm. The larger cells show vesicular nuclei with prominent nucleoli (ISUP grades 2 or 3) and can be quite similar to the most common cell type seen in tumors with *TFE3* fusion transcripts, whereas the smaller cells show denser chromatin (Fig. 8.1d). Variable amounts of melanin pigment can be present. The tumor cells are arranged in a predominantly nested or solid architecture with occasional papillary, tubular and glandular structures and frequent entrapment of native parenchyma. The smaller cells can be seen clustered around hyaline globules composed of basement membrane material. Additional morphological features seen in a subset of cases include extensive hyalinization, pure papillary morphology, cystic changes, and monophasic neoplasms with clear cell or extensive eosinophilic cytoplasm and solid features [33, 39, 40]. Cases showing significant morphological overlap with tRCC bearing *TFE3* fusion transcripts have also been reported [41].

tRCCs show a characteristic immunohistochemical profile, which can be helpful in establishing their diagnosis. In contrast to other RCC subtypes, tumors with *TFE3* fusion transcripts show none or underexpression of epithelial markers such as cytokeratin subunits and epithelial membrane antigen (EMA), whereas cases with *TFEB* fusion transcripts can show more robust cytokeratin expression [40, 41]. However, similar to other types of RCC, tRCCs with both *TFE3* and *TFEB* fusion transcripts frequently express RCC markers such as CD10 and RCC protein and markers of renal tubular differentiation (Pax8 and Pax2)[40, 42]. The majority of *TFEB* tRCCs show expression of the melanocytic markers Melan-A and HMB-45, which can be also seen in a subset of cases bearing *TFE3* fusions. Cathepsin K is expressed in most cases with *PRCC-TFE3* and *TFEB* fusion transcripts, but not in other types of RCC; however, its usefulness in the diagnosis of tRCC is limited by the lack of expression in tumors with *ASPL-TFE3*, *NONO-TFE3*, and *SFPQ-TFE3* fusions [32, 40, 43]. Finally, immunohistochemical antibodies against TFE3 (Fig. 8.1c) and TFEB proteins have been shown to be sensitive and specific markers for the diagnosis of tRCC [35, 36], in keeping with their expected nuclear overexpression in these tumors. However, their use can be limited by technical challenges resulting in variable staining.

Despite the distinctive morphological features found in the majority of tRCC, the spectrum of changes seen in these tumors is variable, and some degree of overlap with other types of RCC may be occasionally appreciated, especially clear cell and papillary RCC. The use of a panel of immunohistochemical antibodies as discussed above can be helpful in these scenarios. As an important observation, nuclear TFE3 and TFEB immunohistochemical expression should be interpreted in the appropriate morphological and immunophenotypical context, as other types of RCC have been shown to overexpress these markers and additional mechanisms of *TFE3* and *TFEB* activation, including gene amplification, have been documented in the absence of gene rearrangements [44–47]. Recently, *TFE3* gene rearrangements, including identical fusion transcripts as described in tRCC, have been identified in a subset of renal perivascular epithelioid cell tumors (PEComas), and some degree of morphological overlap between these tumors and tRCC can also be appreciated [32].

8.5 Staging and Surgical Considerations

The staging for translocation renal cell carcinoma (RCC) follows the same tumor, node, metastasis (TNM) and group staging system used by the American Joint Committee on Cancer (AJCC) for all types of RCC [48]. As part of the full initial staging, this requires preoperative imaging and thorough intraoperative assessment of the extent of disease. For complete preoperative staging, the imaging, at a minimum, includes cross-sectional imaging of the chest (CT), abdomen, and pelvis (MR or CT). Additional imaging such as brain MRI or bone scans are generally reserved only for those patients with signs or symptoms of such involvement.

Intraoperatively, in addition to complete resection of the tumor, attention should be paid to the regional lymph nodes to determine the potential of locoregional spread. Lymph node mapping studies indicate that these anatomic templates are, for the right kidney, paracaval, precaval, retrocaval, and interaortocaval lymph nodes and, for the left kidney, para-aortic, preaortic, retroaortic, and interaortocaval lymph nodes [49, 50].

The surgical approach to tRCC largely mirrors the surgical approach to RCC in general. In terms of technical considerations, whether this be a partial nephrectomy or radical nephrectomy and whether approached as an open or minimally invasive surgery, a complete surgical resection with negative margins is the primary goal. Due to the relative rarity of tRCC, there are few reports about the specific surgical issues in this population.

For those primary renal lesions <4 cm and confined to the kidney (T1a), a nephron-sparing surgical approach with partial nephrectomy is reasonable if the lesion can be completely resected with negative margins [51]. While there are very few large series specifically focused on patients with tRCC, it does appear that a higher proportion of such patients are treated with radical nephrectomy when compared to the general population of those with RCC, even in the T1 setting [5, 10, 52]. However, this may be a reflection of the fact that the tRCC population tends to present at more advanced stage compared with non-translocation RCC [5, 52]. A recent report on 56 children, adolescents, and young adults with tRCC noted that greater than 60% had Stage 3 or 4 disease, and of those with pathologic evaluation of lymph nodes, over 66% had lymph nodes involved [5]. Additionally, there was no difference in the median size of tumors with or without LN involvement (6.5 cm vs. 6.7 cm, respectively). This speaks to the fact that regardless of the surgical approach to the primary tumor, either partial or radical nephrectomy and either open or minimally invasive surgery, regional lymph nodes should be removed when tRCC is suspected. Some authors have suggested that aggressive lymphadenectomy may improve outcomes in patients with tRCC as there are reported to be a higher than expected rate of long-term survivors with nodal involvement. However, such reports are small retrospective series and data collected from administrative databases [16, 53, 54].

In addition to regional lymph node dissection, other adjunctive surgical resection may include addressing a venous tumor thrombus or the setting of resectable metastatic disease (metastectomy). The limited data available would indicate that similar to non-translocation RCC, approximately 5–10% of tRCC cases will have venous tumor thrombi [5]. The surgical approach to such cases should mirror that of the general approach to RCC with venous extension. Complete excision of all tumor should be the goal, and this can reasonably be accomplished with a multidisciplinary surgical team when such adjuncts as complete hepatic mobilization or intrathoracic access (+/− cardiopulmonary bypass) are required. Multiple published series demonstrate the safety and efficacy of such an approach [55–57].

The role of metastectomy for tRCC is unclear. Extrapolating from general RCC reports, Thomas et al. have recently described the M.D. Anderson experience with surgical excision of retroperitoneal recurrences and report 40% remained without evidence of disease at a median of 32 months after resection [58]. Similarly, there are reports of up to 40% long-term survival after metastectomy with a better prognosis for those with first-time, solitary, non-brain metastasis [59]. While the prognosis for tRCC may be considered overall "worse" than more common (ccRCC) RCC variants, judicious use of metastectomy on a case-by-case basis, analogous to practices adopted for other variants of RCC, seems appropriate.

8.6   Systemic Therapy

Despite typical advance stage at presentation, often aggressive behavior, and apparent increasing awareness and diagnosis of tRCC, no formal treatment recommendations are available, as no dedicated powered prospective therapeutic trials have been conducted. Biological targets of interest include c-Met [18, 24, 60], VEGFR, mTOR [8, 61, 62], and PD1/PDL1 immune checkpoint inhibition strategies [63]. Unfortunately, Phase II study of the c-MET inhibitor tivantinib did not produce responses in six tRCC patients treated, and more recent mTOR inhibitor trials (everolimus; ESPN trial) also failed to demonstrate any benefit in seven tRCC patients treated [60, 64].

Evidence of response of tRCCs to VEGF RTKIs is growing, with objective responses and rare durable complete remissions, in both Paediatric and adult patients [9, 61, 65–70]. Malouf et al. report first-line therapy with sunitinib for tRCC achieving a median PFS of 8.2 months ($n = 11$) versus 2 months for cytokines ($n = 9$) (log-rank $p = 0.003$) [61]. Such limited data was extrapolated via retrospective reviews with varying selection criteria and has not been consistently reproduced. Choueiri et al. report a retrospective review of 15 adult tRCC patients treated with anti-VEGF-based therapy (sunitinib, 10; sorafenib, 3; monoclonal anti-VEGF antibodies, 2) and demonstrate 3 objective responses (20%), 7 with disease stabilization (47%), and 5 with progressive disease (33%) [9].

Second-generation more specific and potent VEGF RTKIs are demonstrating promising clinical benefit and diminished off-target effects. Axitinib (INLYTA) is a small molecule inhibitor of VEGFRs 1–3, FDA approved in January 2012 for advanced RCC after failure of one prior systemic therapy. Mechanistically, axitinib is a small molecule adenosine triphosphate (ATP)-competitive inhibitor that binds to the unphosphorylated "DFG-out" conformation of the catalytic domain of RTKs. The unique binding mode in the kinase domain affords its selectivity and relative high potency for VEGFRs 1–3. Clinically, axitinib is the first VEGFR TKI to show superior activity when randomized against another VEGFR TKI (sorafenib) in a pivotal Phase III RCC trial (AXIS trial), though tRCC was not studied [71].

Recent reports of possibly improved durable response rates using immune checkpoint inhibitor therapy for RCC [63, 72, 73], compared with historical data with cytokines, and FDA approval of several such inhibitors [63, 65], have propelled PD1/PDL1 immune checkpoint inhibitor therapy to the forefront of much RCC-based clinical investigation. The PD-L1 ligand is not expressed in a normal kidney but is expressed in many RCC specimens, including tRCC [63]. Interestingly, PD-L1 tumor expression is associated with a worse clinical outcome, in general, and shorter OS in RCC patients treated with anti-VEGF RTKIs [74].

Recently, Motzer et al. published the results of a Phase II trial of the PD1 inhibitor nivolumab in metastatic RCC, demonstrating an objective response rate of 20, 22, and 20% and median OS of 18.2, 25.5, and 24.7 months for doses 0.3, 2, and 10 mg/kg given intravenously every 3 weeks, respectively. Responses were noted more commonly in PD-L1 expressing tumors ($\geq$ 5% PD-L1 expression) with ORR of 31%, but ORR of 18% of tumors expressing <5% PD-L1 are still among the best ORR in RCC. Median OS was not reached in PD-L1 $\geq$ 5% group and 18.2 months in the PD-L1 <5% group, the latter similar to that achieved with axitinib therapy in the second-line setting [72]. Some responding patients continued to respond for nearly a year after cessation of therapy [73]. Nivolumab received its FDA approval for treatment of patients with RCC failing after prior anti-VEGF-based therapy in November 2015.

Pembrolizumab, the first FDA-approved PD1 inhibitor (September 2014), [75] similarly, is a humanized monoclonal antibody with potent and selective inhibition of PD1 and is now being investigated in Paediatrics (NCT02332668) and in RCC both alone (NCT02212730) and in combination with axitinib (NCT02133742), pazopanib (NCT02014636), and ipilimumab or interferon-α (NCT02089685).

Importantly and relevant to tRCC studies in development, Atkins et al. recently reported preliminary results of study NCT02133742 [76]. On this study, axitinib is administered orally 5 mg twice daily, and pembrolizumab is administered 2 mg/kg intravenously on day 1 of each 3-week cycle. As of March 1, 2016, 52 patients (79% male, 87% white, mean age 61 years) were enrolled. Eleven (21.2%) patients discontinued both treatments: disease progression ($n = 4$), treatment-emergent AEs ($n = 6$; diarrhea, headache/joint pain, fatigue/joint pain, colitis/hepatitis, aggravated rheumatoid arthritis/psoriasis, and drug-induced liver injury), and others ($n = 1$). Thirty-five (67.3%) patients had objective response: 2 had complete response and 33 had partial responses; 11 patients had stable disease. Most common (>2 patients) grade 3 AEs included hypertension ($n = 10$), diarrhea, headache, hyponatremia, alanine aminotransferase (ALT) increased, and aspartate aminotransferase (AST) increased ($n = 3$ each). Grade 4 AEs included dyspnea and hyperuricemia ($n = 1$ each). Immune-related $\geq$ grade 3 AEs included ALT and AST ($n = 2$ each) and diarrhea and colitis ($n = 1$ each). This preliminary analysis indicates axitinib plus pembrolizumab is well tolerated and exhibits antitumor activity in treatment-naïve patients with clear cell RCC.

8.7 Future Directions: Trials AREN03B2, AREN14B1-Q, and AREN1621

The Children's Oncology Group had advanced a biology, tumor banking, and risk stratification study for all Paediatric, adolescent, and young adult patients with renal tumors (AREN03B2). As of 2016, 212 patients with RCC had enrolled, including 88 tRCC, all from patients <30 years of age and >90% from patients <21 years of age. Such cases have all been centrally reviewed by three pathologists and have been subject to the diagnostic molecular scrutiny mentioned above. Pathological details have now been reported [77]. In addition, study AREN14B1-Q will focus on platform-based genomic interrogation of both RNA and DNA from 60 of these tRCC, including whole genome sequencing. Such investigations hold promise to expand our current molecular and pathologic understanding of tRCC in younger patients.

More recently, study AREN1721 is set to launch in August, 2018, a trial comparing axitinib vs nivolumab vs their combination in patients with advanced tRCC for patients of all ages, a collaboration between the Children's Oncology Group and adult oncology cooperative groups, to operate through the National Cancer Trials Network. Such study will be the first dedicated study of tRCC and benchmark the clinical behavior of tRCC across all age groups, as well as any clinical benefit of anti-angiogenic and immune checkpoint inhibitor therapy. An additional tumor bank will be created as part of this study, facilitating further biologic investigation, ultimately with the goal to identify and refine novel targeted therapy for patients with tRCC.

References

1. Argani P, Ladanyi M. Translocation carcinomas of the kidney. Clin Lab Med. 2005;25:363–78.
2. Argani P. The evolving story of renal translocation carcinoma. Am J Clin Pathol. 2006;126: 332–4. Comment on: Am J Clin Pathol. 2006; 26:349–364
3. Ramphal R, Pappo A, Zielenska M, Grant R, Ngan BY. Pediatric renal cell carcinoma: clinical, pathologic, and molecular abnormalities associated with the members of the Mit transcription factor family. Am J Clin Pathol. 2006;126:349–64.
4. Geller JI, Argani P, Adeniran A, et al. Translocation renal cell carcinoma: lack of negative impact due to lymph node spread. Cancer. 2008;112:1607–16.
5. Geller JI, Ehrlich PF, Cost NG, et al. Characterization of adolescent and pediatric renal cell carcinoma: a report from the Children's oncology group study AREN03B2. Cancer. 2015;121(14):2457–64.
6. Ehrlich PF, Cost NG, Khanna G, et al. A description of the surgical experience in children, adolescents and young adults with renal cell carcinoma: a report from the Children's oncology group study AREN 03B2. BJU Int. 2012;110.(Supplement 2:18.
7. Zhong M, De Angelo P, Osborne L, et al. Translocation renal cell carcinomas in adults: a single-institution experience. Am J Surg Pathol. 2012;36(5):654–62.
8. Kauffman E, Gupta G, Cecchi F, et al. Characterization of the Akt-mTOR pathway in TFE3-fusion renal cell cancers and implications for targeted therapy. Dent Abstr. 2012;448
9. Choueiri TK, Lim ZD, Hirsch MS, et al. Vascular endothelial growth factor-targeted therapy for the treatment of adult metastatic Xp11.2 translocation renal cell carcinoma. Cancer. 2010;116(22):5219–25.
10. Malouf GG, Camparo P, Molinié V, et al. Transcription factor E3 and transcription factor EB renal cell carcinomas: clinical features, biological behavior and prognostic factors. J Urol. 2011;185(1):24–9. Epub 2010 Nov 12
11. Camparo P, Vasiliu V, Molinie V, et al. Renal translocation carcinomas – Clinicopathologic, Immunohistochemical, and gene expression profiling, analysis of 31 cases with a review of the literature. Am J Surg Pathol. 2008;35:656–70.
12. Meyer PN, Clark JI, Flanigan RC, et al. Xp11.2 translocation renal cell carcinoma with very aggressive course in five adults. Am J Clin Pathol. 2007;128(1):70–9.
13. Hung CC, Pan CC, Lin CC, et al. Xp11.2 translocation renal cell carcinoma: clinical experience of Taipei Veterans General Hospital. J Chin Med Assoc. 2011;74(11):500–4.
14. Dal Cin P, Stas M, Sciot R, De Wever I, Van Damme B, Van den Berghe H. Translocation (X;1) reveals metastasis 31 years after renal cell carcinoma. Cancer Genet Cytogenet. 1998;101:58–61.
15. Arnoux V, Long JA, Fiard G, et al. Xp11.2 translocation renal carcinoma in adults over 50 years of age: about four cases. Prog Urol. 2012;22(15):932–7.
16. Geller J, Khoury J, and Dome J. Author's Reply re: Letter to the Editor re: 'Geller J and Dome J. Lymph node involvement does not predict poor outcome in pediatric renal cell carcinoma. Cancer. October 1, 2004;101:1575–1583.' Cancer 2005; 103(6):1318.
17. Aoyagi T, Shinohara N, Kubota-Chikai K, et al. Long-term survival in a patient with node-positive adult-onset Xp11.2 translocation renal cell carcinoma. Urol Int. 2011;86(4):487–90.
18. Hemesath TJ, Steingrimsson E, McGill G, et al. Microphthalmia, a critical factor in melanocyte development, defines a discrete transcription factor family. Genes Dev. 1994;8:2770–80.
19. Hodgkinson CA, Moore KJ, Nakayama A, et al. Mutations at the mouse microphthalmia locus are associated with defects in a gene encoding a novel basic-helix-loop-helix-zipper protein. Cell. 1993;74:395–404.
20. Yasumoto K, Mahalingam H, Suzuki H, Yoshizawa M, Yokoyama K. Transcriptional activation of the melanocyte-specific genes by the human homolog of the mouse microphthalmia protein. J Biochem. 1995;118:874–81.

21. Weterman AJ, van Groningen JJM, Jansen A, van Kessel AG. Nuclear localization and transactivating capacities of the papillary renal cell carcinoma-associated TFE3 and PRCC (fusion) proteins. Oncogene. 2000;19:69–74.
22. Kuiper RP, Schepens M, Thijssen J, et al. Upregulation of the transcription factor TFEB in t(6;11)(p21;q13)-positive renal cell carcinoma due to promoter substitution. Hum Mol Genet. 2003;12:1661–9.
23. Medendorp K, van Groningen JJM, Schepens M, et al. Molecular mechanisms underlying the MiT translocation subgroup of renal cell carcinomas. Cytogenet Genome Res. 2007;118:157–65.
24. Tsuda M, Davis IJ, Argani P, et al. TFE3 fusions activate MET signaling by transcriptional up-regulation, defining another class of tumors as candidates for therapeutic MET inhibition. Cancer Res. 2007;67:919–29.
25. McGill GG, Horstmann M, Widlund HR, et al. Bcl2 regulation by the melanocyte master regulator Mitf modulates lineage survival and melanoma cell viability. Cell. 2002;109:707–18.
26. Du J, Widlund HR, Hartsmann MA, et al. Critical role of CDK2 for melanoma growth linked to its melanocyte-specific transcriptional regulation by MITF. Cancer Cell. 2004;6:565–76.
27. Busca R, Berra E, Gaggioli C, et al. Hypoxia-inducible factor 1α is a new target of microphthalmia-associated transcription factor (MITF) in melanoma cells. J Cell Biol. 2005;170:49–59.
28. Nijman SMB, Hijmans EM, El Messaoudi S, van Dongen MMW, Sardet C, Bernards R. A functional genetic screen identifies TFE3 as a gene that confers resistance to the antiproliferative effects of the retinoblastoma protein and transforming growth factor-β. J Biol Chem. 2006;281:21582–7.
29. Waterman MAJ, van Groningen JJM, Tertoolen L, van Kessel AG. Impairment of MAD2B-PRCC interaction in mitotic checkpoint defective t(X;1)-positive renal cell carcinomas. PNAS. 2001;98:13808–13.
30. Mathur M, Samuels HH. Role of PSF-TFE3 oncoprotein in the development of papillary renal cell carcinomas. Oncogene. 2007;26:277–83.
31. Ladanyi M, Lui MY, Antonescu CR, et al. The der(17)t(X;17)(p11;q25) of human alveolar soft part sarcoma fuses the TFE3 transcription factor gene to ASPL, a novel gene at 17q25. Oncogene. 2001;20:48–57.
32. Argani P, Zhong M, Reuter VE, et al. TFE3-fusion variant analysis defines specific clinicopathologic associations among Xp11 translocation cancers. Am J Surg Pathol. 2016;40:723–37.
33. Rao Q, Liu B, Cheng L, et al. A clinicopathologic study emphasizing unusual morphology, novel alpha-TFEB gene fusion point, immunobiomarkers, and ultrastructural features, as well as detection of the gene fusion by fluorescence in situ hybridization. Am J Surg Pathol. 2012;36:1327–38.
34. Green WM, Yonescu R, Morsberger L, et al. Utilization of a TFE3 break-apart FISH assay in a renal tumor consultation service. Am J Surg Pathol. 2013;37:1150–63.
35. Argani P, Lal P, Hutchinson B, Lui MY, Reuter VE, Ladanyi M. Aberrant nuclear immunoreactivity for TFE3 in neoplasms with TFE3 gene fusions. Am J Surg Pathol. 2003;27:750–61.
36. Argani P, Lae M, Hutchinson B, et al. Renal carcinomas with the t (6;11)(p21;q12). Clinicopathologic features and demonstration of the specific alpha-TFEB gene fusion by immunohistochemistry, RT-PCR and DNA PCR. Am J Surg Pathol. 2005;29:230–40.
37. Malouf GG, Su X, Gao J, et al. Next-generation sequencing of translocation renal cell carcinoma reveals novel RNA splicing patterns and frequent mutations of chromatin-remodeling genes. Clin Cancer Res. 2014;20:4129–40.
38. Argani P. MiT family translocation renal cell carcinoma. Semin Diagn Pathol. 2015;32:103–13.
39. Inamura K, Fujiwara M, Togashi Y, et al. Diverse fusion patterns and heterogeneous clinicopathologic features of renal cell carcinoma with t(6;11) translocation. Am J Surg Pathol. 2012;36:35–42.
40. Argani P, Yonescu R, Morsberger L, et al. Molecular confirmation of t(6;11)(p21;q12) renal cell carcinoma in archival paraffin-embedded material using a break-apart TFEB FISH assay expands its clinicopathologic spectrum. Am J Surg Pathol. 2012;36:1516–26.

41. Smith NE, Illei PB, Allaf M, et al. T(6;11) renal cell carcinoma (RCC) expanded immuno-histochemical profile emphasizing novel RCC markers and report of 10 new genetically confirmed cases. Am J Surg Pathol. 2014;38:604–14.
42. Argani P, Hicks J, De Marzo AM, et al. Xp11 translocation renal cell carcinoma (RCC): extended immunohistochemical profile emphasizing novel RCC markers. Am J Surg Pathol. 2010;34:1295–303.
43. Martignoni G, Gobbo S, Camparo P, et al. Differential expression of cathepsin K in neoplasms harboring TFE3 gene fusions. Mod Pathol. 2011;24:1313–9.
44. Hong SB, Oh HB, Valera VA, Baba M, Schmidt LS, Linehan WM. Inactivation of the FLCN tumor suppressor gene induces TFE3 transcriptional activity by increasing its nuclear localization. PLoS One. 2010;5(12):e15793.
45. Macher-Goeppinger S, Roth W, Wagener N, et al. Molecular heterogeneity of TFE3 activation in renal cell carcinomas. Mod Pathol. 2012;25:308–15.
46. Cajaiba MM, Jennings LJ, Rohan SM, et al. ALK-rearranged renal cell carcinomas in children. Genes Chromosomes Cancer. 2016;55:442–51.
47. Argani P, Reuter VE, Zhang L, et al. TFEB-amplified renal cell carcinomas: an aggressive molecular subset demonstrating variable melanocytic marker expression and morphologic heterogeneity. Am J Surg Pathol. 2016;40:1484–95.
48. Edge SB, Byrd DR, Compton CC, et al. AJCC Cancer staging manual. 7th ed. New York: Springer-Verlag; 2010.
49. Crispen PL, Breau RH, Allmer C, et al. Lymph node dissection at the time of radical nephrectomy for high-risk clear cell renal cell carcinoma: indications and recommendations for surgical templates. Eur Urol. 2011;59:18–23.
50. Capitanio U, Becker F, Blute ML, et al. Lymph node dissection in renal cell carcinoma. Eur Urol. 2011;60:1212–20.
51. Gorin MA, Ball MW, Pierorazio PM, et al. Partial nephrectomy for the treatment of translocation renal cell carcinoma. Clin Genitourin Cancer. 2015;13:e199–201.
52. Xu L, Yang R, Gan W, et al. Xp11.2 translocation renal cell carcinomas in young adults. BMC Urol. 2015;15:57.
53. Indolfi P, Bisogno G, Cecchetto G, et al. Local lymph node involvement in pediatric renal cell carcinoma: a report from the Italian TREP project. Pediatr Blood Cancer. 2008;51:475–8.
54. Rialon KL, Gulack BC, Englum BR, et al. Factors impacting survival in children with renal cell carcinoma. J Pediatr Surg. 2015;50:1014–8.
55. Karnes RJ, Blute ML. Surgery insight: management of renal cell carcinoma with associated inferior vena cava thrombus. Nat Clin Pract Urol. 2008;5:329–39.
56. Klatte T, Pantuck AJ, Riggs SB, et al. Prognostic factors for renal cell carcinoma with tumor thrombus extension. J Urol. 2007;178:1189–95. discussion 1195
57. Gayed BA, Youssef R, Darwish O, et al. Multi-disciplinary surgical approach to the management of patients with renal cell carcinoma with venous tumor thrombus: 15 year experience and lessons learned. BMC Urol. 2016;16:43.
58. Thomas AZ, Adibi M, Borregales LD, et al. Surgical Management of Local Retroperitoneal Recurrence of renal cell carcinoma after radical nephrectomy. J Urol. 2015;194:316–22.
59. Kavolius JP, Mastorakos DP, Pavlovich C, et al. Resection of metastatic renal cell carcinoma. J Clin Oncol Off J Am Soc Clin Oncol. 1998;16:2261–6.
60. Wagner AJ, Goldberg JM, Dubois SG, et al. Tivantinib (ARQ 197), a selective inhibitor of mesenchymal-epithelial transition factor, in patients with microphthalmia transcription factor-associated tumors: Results of a multicenter phase 2 trial. Cancer. 2012 May 17. (epub ahead of print).
61. Malouf GG, Camparo P, Oudard S, et al. Targeted agents in metastatic Xp11 translocation/TFE3 gene fusion renal cell carcinoma (RCC): a report from the juvenile RCC network. Ann Oncol. 2010;21(9):1834–8. Epub 2010 Feb 12
62. Parikh J, Coleman T, Messias N, Brown J. Temsirolimus in the treatment of renal cell carcinoma associated with Xp11.2 translocation/TFE gene fusion proteins: a case report and review of literature. Rare Tumors. 2009;1(2):e53.

63. Massari F, Santoni M, Ciccarese C, et al. PD-1 blockade therapy in renal cell carcinoma: current studies and future promises. Cancer Treat Rev. 2015;41:114–21.
64. Tannir NM, Jonasch E, et al. Everolimus versus sunitinib prospective evaluation in metastatic non-clear cell renal cell carcinoma (the ESPN trial): a multicenter randomized phase 2 trial. J Clin Oncol. 2014;32:5s. suppl; abstr 4505
65. Liu YC, Chang PM, Liu CY, et al. Sunitinib-induced nephrotic syndrome in association with drug response in a patient with Xp11. 2 translocation renal cell carcinoma. Jpn J Clin Oncol. 2011;41(11):1277–81. Epub 2011 Sep 29
66. Numakura K, Tsuchiya N, Yuasa T, et al. A case study of metastatic Xp11.2 translocation renal cell carcinoma effectively treated with sunitinib. Int J Clin Oncol. 2011;16(5):577–80. Epub 2010 Dec 15
67. Hou MM, Hsieh JJ, Chang NJ, et al. Response to sorafenib in a patient with metastatic xp11 translocation renal cell carcinoma. Clin Drug Investig. 2010;30(11):799–804.
68. Pwint TP, Macaulay V, Roberts IS, Sullivan M, Protheroe A. An adult Xp11.2 translocation renal carcinoma showing response to treatment with sunitinib. Urol Oncol. 2011;29(6):821–4. Epub 2009 Dec 4
69. Choueiri TK, Mosquera JM, Hirsch MS. A case of adult metastatic Xp11 translocation renal cell carcinoma treated successfully with sunitinib. Clin Genitourin Cancer. 2009;7(3):E93–4.
70. Chowdhury T, Prchard-Jones K, Sebire NJ, et al. Persistent complete response after single-agent Sunitinib treatment in a case of TFE translocation positive relapsed metastatic pediatric renal cell carcinoma. J Pediatr Hematol Oncol. 2013;35(1):e1–3.
71. Rini BI, Escudier B, Tomczak P, et al. Comparative effectiveness of axitinib versus sorafenib in advanced renal cell carcinoma (AXIS): a randomised phase 3 trial. Lancet. 2011;378:1931–9.
72. Motzer RJ, Rini BI, McDermott DF, et al. Nivolumab for metastatic renal cell carcinoma: results of a randomized phase II trial. J Clin Oncol. 2015;33(13):1430–7.
73. McDermott DF, Drake CG, Sznol M, et al. Survival, durable response, and long-term safety in patients with previously treated advanced renal cell carcinoma receiving Nivolumab. J Clin Oncol. 2015;33(18):2013–20.
74. Brunot A, Bernhard J-C, Yacoub M, et al. PDL-1 and PDL1 expressions in clear cell renal cell carcinoma (ccRCC) of metastatic patients with sunitinib first-line treatment. J Clin Oncol. 2015;33:15. suppl; abstr e14002
75. Faghfuri E, Faramarzi MA, Nikfar S, Abdollahi M. Nivolumab and pembrolizumab as immune-modulating monoclonal antibodies targeting the PD-1 receptor to treat melanoma. Expert Rev Anticancer Ther. 2015;15(9):981–93.
76. Atkins MB, Choueiri TK, Hodi S, et al. Pembrolizumab (MK-3475) plus low-dose ipilimumab (IPI) in patients (pts) with advanced melanoma (MEL) or renal cell carcinoma (RCC): data from the KEYNOTE-029 phase 1 study. J Clin Oncol. 2015;33:3009. suppl; abstr 3009
77. Cajaiba MM, Dyer LM, Geller JI, Jennings LJ, George D, Kirschmann D, Rohan SM, Cost NG, Khanna G, Mullen EA, Dome JS, Fernandez CV, Perlman EJ. The classification of pediatric and young adult renal cell carcinomas registered on the Children's Oncology Group (COG) protocol AREN03B2 after focused genetic testing. Cancer. 2018; https://doi.org/10.1002/cncr.31578. [Epub ahead of print]

Renal Cell Carcinoma with Sarcomatoid Features

Borchiellini Delphine, Ambrosetti Damien, and Barthélémy Philippe

9.1 Introduction

Histological features of renal cell carcinomas (RCC) have been described and enriched over the past decades, and the World Health Organization (WHO) classification recognizes several now well-known subtypes like clear-cell, papillary, and chromophobe carcinomas. The characterization of RCC is still evolving, since the 2016 edition of the WHO classification mentions 14 different histologic subtypes [1].

One particular entity remains to be better characterized, RCC with sarcomatoid differentiation (sRCC), corresponding to morphologic sarcoma-like characteristics. This differentiation is not considered anymore as a distinct subtype of RCC but can be identified as a component of all clear-cell and non-clear-cell RCC. It has been detected in up to 10% of clear-cell (cc), chromophobe (chr), and unclassified RCC, and less frequently in papillary (pap) histology [2, 3].

Weisel et al. firstly described in 1943 a specific entity named as kidney sarcoma [4]. The literature was then enriched with the description of several other cases of sarcomas or sarcomatoid malignant tumors of the kidney that were considered as rare but particularly aggressive malignancies [5]. In the next two decades, a histological variant of sarcomatoid carcinoma of the kidney was described [6]. Many pathologists tended to identify this type of sarcomatoid component associated with every histologic subtype of RCC. At the same time, sarcomatoid differentiation was related to some chromosomal rearrangements and was finally not considered anymore as a specific subtype in the 1997 UICC and AJCC

B. Delphine (✉)
Oncology Department, Antoine Lacassagne Cancer Center, Nice, France
e-mail: Delphine.BORCHIELLINI@nice.unicancer.fr

A. Damien
Pathology Department, Pasteur University Hospital, Nice, France

B. Philippe
Medical Oncology Department, Strasbourg University Hospital, Strasbourg, France

© Springer Nature Switzerland AG 2019
G. G. Malouf, N. M. Tannir (eds.), *Rare Kidney Tumors*,
https://doi.org/10.1007/978-3-319-96989-3_9

classification [7]. This definition was confirmed in the 2004 WHO classification, which recommended to classify sRCC according to the underlying histologic subtype [8].

Delahunt et al. first concluded that genetic and morphologic evidence indicated that sRCC resulted from the final common dedifferentiation of renal epithelial malignancy [9]. More recently, it was suggested that sarcomatoid ccRCC morphologically and immunohistochemically may represent a completed epithelial-mesenchymal transition of ccRCC [10].

If the underlying mechanisms of sarcomatoid dedifferentiation still remain unclear, it is now admitted that sarcomatoid component is an aggressive component that can be part of any localized or advanced clear-cell or non-clear-cell RCC, systematically leading to a poor prognosis, and considered for this reason as a clinical specific entity.

9.2   Pathologic Features

9.2.1   Macroscopic Findings

Primary RCC tumors with sarcomatoid component are rather large, 10 cm in average diameter [11]. The cut surface is often described as soft, fleshy, and gray white, with infiltrative margins. The sarcomatoid component often clearly appears distinct from the associated differentiated component.

9.2.2   Microscopic Findings

Sarcomatoid features are histologically defined as a dedifferentiated tumor with morphologic sarcoma-like characteristics. A sarcomatoid tumor consists of atypical fusiform cells, miming any type of sarcoma. Most often, the morphology is that of the fibrosarcoma, with intersecting fascicles of malignant spindle cells. Heterologous differentiation of osteoid type, chondroid, or rhabdoid is rare. These different aspects can be exclusive or coexist.

Sarcomatoid component is found in a histologically biphasic tumor associated with a differentiated epithelial component defining a typical carcinoma. In this case, it is not a specific type of RCC, as these morphological changes can be found in all subtypes of RCC. The amount of sarcomatoid modification in the RCC has been reported in the literature to vary from 1% to 100%, with a mean and median of ~40%–50%. According to the recommendations of the International Society of Urological Pathology (ISUP), a sarcomatoid component is taken into account regardless of its proportion within the entire tumor [12]. There is no recommendation to quantify this proportion. Sarcomatoid and carcinoma areas may be interwoven or clearly demarcated.

According to the ISUP recommendations, the presence of a sarcomatoid component systematically refers to a grade 4 of Fuhrman classification [12], even if several authors suggest that sRCC has a more aggressive clinical behavior than grade 4 tumors without sarcomatoid component, as well as distinct biological and molecular characteristics [13]. Hence they suggest to describe the sarcomatoid features independently of the grade or, at least, to systematically stipulate the presence of a sarcomatoid component in addition to the grade.

A pure sRCC is defined as an epithelial renal tumor entirely composed of sarcomatoid cells. These tumors are rare, standing for about 5% of all sarcomatoid carcinomas [14]. According to the WHO classification, pure sarcomatoid tumors should be referred as unclassified RCC.

The diagnosis of biphasic sRCC does not require further exploration for histological analysis. In the case of pure sRCC, the diagnosis can be confirmed by additional tests. The epithelial and mesenchymal markers by immunohistochemistry can help to distinguish sRCC from sarcoma. Sarcomatoid component is positive for cytokeratin, and more rarely vimentin. Mesenchymal tissue and sarcoma markers, such as desmin and actin, are rarely expressed in sRCC. Moreover, sarcomatoid areas associated with ccRCC retain high expression of the HIF pathway markers (VEGF, GLUT1, CAIX) [15].

9.2.3 Differential Diagnosis

By definition, sRCC displays similar characteristics as sarcomas. However, some differences help the pathologist to distinguish these two types of tumors. The identification of any RCC subtype within the tumor will eliminate primary renal sarcoma. Renal sarcomas are rare in adults, mainly represented by leiomyosarcomas. Smooth muscular aspects are rarely seen in sRCC.

Undifferentiated and sarcomatous form of urothelial carcinoma can also mimic sRCC. An exhaustive sampling of the tumor can help, by detecting a usual area of urothelial carcinoma.

9.2.4 Epithelial-Mesenchymal Transition

Sarcomatoid tumors and contingents are thought to be derived from the clonal expansion of a subpopulation of neoplastic cells coming from a conventional RCC. There are cellular changes, a metaplastic process in which the tumor cells lose their epithelial characteristics and gain a mesenchymal phenotype. This process is found in other tumor models and is called epithelial–mesenchymal transition (EMT). This change is accompanied by a modification of the cellular characteristics, these being more aggressive because of their increased ability to migrate and metastasize. On the molecular level, there is in particular initially an increase in the expression of Snail and N-cadherin during the initiation of the EMT, before the morphological phenotypic mesenchymal expression [16]. Then other molecular mechanisms are involved, loss of E-cadherin, release of β-catenin into the cytoplasm, and expression of Sparc.

9.2.5 Molecular Alterations

The genetic exploration of these tumors can help for the diagnosis but also to better understand their pathogenesis. Bi et al. performed exome sequencing of matched normal-carcinomatous-sarcomatoid specimens from 21 subjects and showed that sarcomatoid contingents had more somatic mutations [17]. In particular, homozygous mutations in TP53 and BRCA1-associated protein-1 (BAP1) were specifically found in sarcomatoid elements, even if mutually exclusive. This strongly suggests these genes are involved in the evolution toward a sarcomatoid tumor. Moreover, the sarcomatoid and conventional clear-cell carcinomatous elements shared 42% of the somatic single-nucleotide variants (SSNV), mostly in the genes known to be involved in the oncogenesis of ccRCCs (e.g., VHL). More SSNV were observed in sarcomatoid tumors. These results are further proof that the sarcomatoid contingent is derived from conventional ccRCC, after dedifferentiation. Ito et al. performed a genomic copy number analysis in 81 RCC including 17 with sRCC. Sarcomatoid carcinomas showed significantly higher copy number changes (including losses of 9q, 15q, 18p/q, and 22q and gains of 1q and 8q) than ccRCC, papRCC, or chrRCC subtypes [18]. Malouf et al. conducted genomic profiling on paired epithelial and sarcomatoid areas of three sRCC cases. Genomic profiling was performed on another 23 sRCC patients harboring diverse epithelial components. The authors showed on the one hand the existence of genomic characteristics common to the two cell populations, but also specific and recurrent driver mutations in sRCC, including TP53 and NF2 [19]. All these results converge and show a clear lineage between sarcomatoid carcinomas and tumors from which they derive, with involvement of specific signaling and oncogenesis pathway.

9.3   Clinical Characteristics

9.3.1   Epidemiology

In the most recent series, as well as in large previous reports, a sarcomatoid component is found in 2 to 10% of RCC [3, 20–23]. A meta-analysis by Vera-Badillo et al. on 49 studies and more than 7000 patients gives an incidence of 2.9% for sarcomatoid component among cc and non-ccRCC [24].

The most frequent underlying histology is clear-cell given the predominance of ccRCC. However, chrRCC are more likely to undergo sarcomatoid change compared with cc and papRCC. Cheville et al. reported a sarcomatoid component in 5.2% (104/1985) of cc, 8.7% (9/103) of chr, and 1.9% (5/270) of pap histology, when de Peralta-Venturina et al. found similar results with 8% of cc, 9% of chr, and 3% of papRCC [3, 23].

9.3.2 Clinical Presentation

Median age at diagnosis varies between 56 and 62 years old [22, 25–27] and did not seem to differ as compared to patients with non-sRCC in a matched-pair analysis published by Brookman-May et al. This was the same for the sex ratio, with about two men for one woman [28].

Sarcomatoid RCC present frequently with a large primitive renal tumor, with a median size between 9 and 10 cm and tumor ≥T3 in more than 70% of the cases [20, 22, 26, 29, 30]. Locoregional lymph node involvement is less frequent, representing usually <25% of the cases [20, 26, 30, 31] except for Pamela et al. who reported an N-positive status in 52% in 23 patients [22]. About 90% of the patients have symptoms at presentation, like abdominal pain or hematuria [29].

In most series, the majority of patients with a sRCC present with a metastatic disease [3, 20, 21, 27, 29, 31–33].

9.3.3 Prognostic Significance of Sarcomatoid Component

As previously described, it is now admitted that sRCC should no longer be considered as separate tumor entity, but a powerful prognostic factor, as cancer-specific survival is uniformly poor for patients whose tumors exhibited sarcomatoid changes, regardless of the underlying histologic subtype, both in the localized and metastatic settings [23, 28, 30, 34].

Cheville et al. showed that even among the subset of patients with grade 4 ccRCCs, the presence of a sarcomatoid component was significantly associated with outcome (risk ratio 1.59; 95% CI 1.12–2.27; $P = 0.010$) [23].

The International Metastatic Renal Cell Carcinoma Database Consortium (IMDC) recently examined 230 sRCC compared with 2056 non-sRCC. Patients with sRCC had significantly worse IMDC prognostic criteria compared with non-sRCC (11% vs. 19% favorable risk; 49% vs. 57% intermediate risk; and 40% vs. 24% poor risk; $P < 0.0001$), as well as a shorter time to relapse and worse clinical outcome with targeted therapy [21]. Nguyen et al. further suggested that histologic subtype impacts cancer-specific survival in sRCC patients treated surgically, as patients with non-cc sRCC had significantly lower CSS than patients with cc sRCC ($p = 0.035$). In multivariable analyses, non-cc sRCC conferred a higher risk of cancer-specific death compared with cc sRCC (HR 2.30, 95% CI 1.38–3.82, $p = 0.001$) [26].

The latest 2016 guidelines from the European Association of Urology (EAU) define the sarcomatoid component as one of the prognostic factors validated by the International Society of Urological Pathology (ISUP) consensus and the new WHO 2016 classification of RCC that has to be reported in routine practice [12, 35].

9.3.3.1 Percentage of Sarcomatoid Component (PSC)

The percentage of sarcomatoid component (PSC) has been mentioned as a potential prognostic indicator for patients both in the localized and the metastatic settings. However, no threshold has been statistically and reproducibly established in the literature [31]. The main studies investigating the prognostic role of PSC are detailed in Table 9.1.

All eight studies were retrospective. Patients were mixed with nonmetastatic (M0) and metastatic (M1) disease. Heterogeneous cut points were considered for PSC. In univariate analysis, PSC was prognostic for survival at specific but different determined cut points (10%, 30%, or 50%) in four studies [3, 27, 31, 36] and as a continuous variable in three studies [20, 33, 36]. However, it was not associated with survival in two studies [30, 37].

In multivariate analysis, PSC remained an independent prognostic factor for survival in only one study by Park et al., with a cut point of 10% [27]. In two other studies, subgroup analysis showed that PSC was a statistically significant factor for M0 patients, in Kim et al. study [20], whereas it was only for M1 patients for Adibi et al. [31].

These conflicting results prevent from any definitive conclusion on the recommended level for PSC significance.

9.4 Treatment

For more than two decades, the poor prognosis of sRCC has been an issue, underlying the unmet need for alternative options of treatment, both in localized and metastatic settings. However, no reel successful strategy has emerged.

9.4.1 Localized Disease

9.4.1.1 Surgery

As previously described, a majority of patients with sRCC initially presents with a metastatic involvement. Thus, most publications investigating outcome or treatment have mixed patients with localized and advanced disease. Only one single-institution retrospective study has evaluated the outcome of 77 localized sRCC after surgical resection with curative intent [30]. A majority of patients had symptoms (91%) and T3/T4 tumor (77%). Only 2 patients had a partial nephrectomy, whereas the 75 remaining patients had radical nephrectomy, with inferior vena cava thrombectomy in 27%. Moreover, 61% had a lymph node dissection and 22% an additional organ resection. Pathological positive lymph nodes, necrosis, and lymphovascular invasion were seen in 25%, 34%, and 19% of the cases, respectively. The characteristics of histologic subtype, PSC, and outcome are detailed in Table 9.1. The median overall survival (OS) was 24 months, and 56/73 patients (72%) experienced a recurrence with a median time of 26.2 months.

Table 9.1 Studies investigating the association between percentage of sarcomatoid component (PSC) cut point and outcome in patients (pts) with sRCC

	N in the total cohort and by stage	Histology subtype	Pts with sRCC	Median PSC	PSC cut point	Median PFS (months)	Median OS (months)	Prognostic factors on OS in univariate analysis	Prognostic factors in multivariate analysis
De Peralta et al. [3]	101 Localized 76 Metastatic 25	Cc 79% Pap 7% Chr 8% Other 6%	All analyzed cohort	40%	<10 11–25 26–50 >50	NA	19	• TNM • 50% PSC • LVI	TNM
Cheville et al. [23]	120 Localized 66 Metastatic 54	Cc 87% Pap 4% Chr 7.5% Other 1.5%	All analyzed cohort	NA	5–10: 44% 15–50: 49% >50: 7%	NA	8	*For CSS* • Distant metastases • Tumor necrosis • Sarcomatoid component (PSC not associated with CSS)	NA but sarcomatoid component associated with outcome after adjusted for TNM, tumor size, and tumor necrosis
Shuch et al. [33]	104 Localized 32 Metastatic 72	Cc 65% Pap 13% Chr 11% Other 11%	All analyzed cohort	50%	<25: 27% 25–50: 15% 50–75: 28% ≥75: 30%	NA	5, 9	• ECOG PS • Tumor size • LVI • Necrosis (by quartile) • PSC (by quartile) • Distant metastases	• ECOG PS • Tumor size • LVI
Park et al.[27]	83 Localized 28 Metastatic 55	NA	40 (48%)	27.5%	<10: 65% ≥10: 35%	12	35	• Time < 1 year from initial diagnosis to TKI initiation • Thrombocytosis • High Fuhrman grade • ≥10% PSC • ≥10% tumor necrosis	• Time < 1 year from initial diagnosis to TKI initiation • ≥10% PSC

(continued)

Table 9.1 (continued)

	N in the total cohort and by stage	Histology subtype	Pts with sRCC	Median PSC	PSC cut point	Median PFS (months)	Median OS (months)	Prognostic factors on OS in univariate analysis	Prognostic factors in multivariate analysis
Kim et al. [20]	55 Localized 26 Metastatic 29	Cc 74.5% Pap 9% Chr 5.5% Other 11%	All analyzed cohort	NA	≤25: 64% 26–50: 16% 50–75: 20%	6	All cohort: 8.7 M0: 21.2 M1: 4	• pT • Tumor size • pN • Distant metastases • PSC (continuous variable)	• pT • Tumor size • Distant metastases • PSC >25% (not in the M1 subgroup)
Zhang et al. [36]	411 pts. with grade 4 RCC Localized 257 Metastatic 154	Cc 85% Pap 4% Chr 6% Other 5%	204 (compared with 207 pts. with non-sRCC)	For 204 pts. with sRCC: 42%	**For 204 pts with sRCC:** <30: 47% ≥30: 53%	NA	**CSS:** 8	**For CSS in 204 pts with sRCC:** • Symptoms at presentation • Tumor size • pT • pN • Distant metastases • Tumor necrosis • Amount of sarcomatoid component (by 10% increase) • PCS ≥30%	**For 411 pts with grade 4 RCC** • Age at surgery • pT • pN • Distant metastases • Tumor necrosis • Sarcomatoid component

| Merrill et al. [30] | 77 | Localized 77 Metastatic 0 | Cc 73% Other 27% | All analyzed cohort | NA | 1–24: 51% 25–49: 12% 50–74: 10% 75–99: 16% | Median time to recurrence: 26.2 | 24 | | • pT4 • pN • LVI | • pT • pN |
| Adibi et al. [31] | 186 | Localized 64 Metastatic 122 | Cc 73% Other 27% | All analyzed cohort | 25% | ≤10: 39% >10: 61% | NA | 12.6 | • PSC >10% (other variables NA) | | • Tumor size • Distant metastases • PSC >40% for M1 patients |

Cc clear-cell, *Chr* chromophobe, *Pap* papillary, *NA* not available, *OS* overall survival, *CSS* cancer-specific survival, *LVI* lymphovascular invasion

9.4.1.2 Adjuvant Treatment

Giving the poor outcome of these patients, the question of adjuvant treatment is rising. In the two published phase 3 trials of adjuvant VEGFR-targeted therapy in RCC, only few patients with sRCC were represented. In the ASSURE trial, the proportion of patients with sarcomatoid features was 8 to 10%, and no specific subgroup analysis has been performed. However, no benefit in disease-free survival was observed with sunitinib or sorafenib versus placebo in all cohorts nor in the very high-risk population [38]. The S-TRAC trial has demonstrated a significant benefit on DFS of adjuvant sunitinib over placebo for high-risk operated localized ccRCC. If its role is still debated, no information is given about sRCC patients [39].

Few data are available on adjuvant radiation therapy (RT) in RCC, and this treatment has not been validated. Eminaga et al. reported a SEER-based study on the role of postoperative RT on survival in sRCC nonmetastatic patients. Among the 314 who had a radical nephrectomy, only 19 (6%) had adjuvant RT. No OS or DFS benefit was observed with RT. Thus, adjuvant (RT) cannot be recommended in sRCC [40].

9.4.2 Metastatic Disease

9.4.2.1 Cytoreductive Nephrectomy

Cytoreductive nephrectomy followed by interferon (IFN) for metastatic RCC showed a survival advantage over IFN alone in two phase 3 trials [41, 42]. However, this benefit has not been confirmed for patients treated with targeted therapies, especially patients with estimated poor outcome [43]. Shuch et al. explored the role of surgery in 62 sRCC metastatic patients, compared to 355 patients with non-sRCC. Despite cytoreductive nephrectomy, sRCC had a dire outcome, leading the authors to conclude that surgery should not be systematically considered up front but reserved to targeted therapy-responding patients [44].

9.4.2.2 Metastasectomy

Local treatment of oligometastatic RCC is a common attitude. Thomas et al. evaluated whether metastasectomy has any survival benefit in patients with metastatic sRCC treated with radical nephrectomy [45]. Among 80 patients with metastasis (56 synchronous and 24 asynchronous), they matched 40 patients that had resection of metastases with 40 patients that did not have metastasectomy. Most patients that underwent metastasectomy had only one metastatic site at the time of surgery (93% in the synchronous group and 100% in the asynchronous group). Patients with brain and bone metastases were more likely to have metastasectomy, but all metastatic sites were represented. Overall survival in patients who underwent metastasectomy for synchronous metastasis compared to nonsurgical patients was 8.4 and 8.0 months ($p = 0.35$), respectively. In the asynchronous group, median OS in the metastasectomy and nonmetastasectomy groups were 36.2 (95% CI 7.6 – not reached) and 13.7 months (95% CI 8.8–41.6, $p = 0.29$). The authors concluded there was no clear survival benefit in sRCC patients who underwent metastasectomy after nephrectomy.

9.4.2.3 Systemic Treatments

Cytokines and Chemotherapy

Giving the poor outcome of sRCC, questions about a specific therapeutic approach for metastatic disease have raised over the past two decades.

Before the era of targeted therapies, cytokines were the standard of care for advanced or metastatic RCC, with limited efficacy and sometimes a difficult to manage toxicity.

Three main clinical trials have demonstrated the PFS benefit of interferon alpha (INFa) associated with bevacizumab [46, 47] and interleukin-2 [48] in the first-line setting. However, no one has included or described the outcome of the specific sRCC subgroup. At the same time, histological similarities with sarcomas have led to evaluate several chemotherapy regimens in sRCC.

Main studies of cytokines or chemotherapy studies specifically dedicated are detailed in Table 9.2.

Most of them are retrospective studies that mixed localized/metastatic sRCC, as well as different histologic subtypes and treatment regimen (cytokines and/or chemotherapy) [32, 49–56]. No prospective study using cytokines has been conducted in sRCC. Retrospective studies on small and heterogeneous cohorts showed variable activity of IFNa or IL2 in sRCC, with OS ranging from 6.5 to 13.8 months [51, 52, 54].

Escudier et al. conducted the first prospective phase 2 study in 2002 in metastatic sRCC. Efficacy and toxicity of a doxorubicin-ifosfamide chemotherapy regimen were assessed in 25 patients with metastatic sRCC. No objective response was observed among the 23 evaluable patients. Survival was short, with a median time to progression (TTP) of 2.2 months and a median OS of 3.9 months. One patient died of toxicity. The results did not support the standard use of doxorubicin–ifosfamide for sRCC [57].

In 2004, Nanus et al. reported the outcome of 18 patients with sRCC ($n = 10$) or rapidly progressing RCC ($n = 8$) treated with doxorubicin–gemcitabine regimen. In sRCC patients, two complete responses were observed, with a TTP of 21 months for one patient and 4 months for the other. One patient had stable disease for 11 months, while TTP was less than 4 months for the seven remaining sRCC patients [53].

Based on these results, two phase 2 prospective studies were conducted. Staehler et al. evaluated this regimen in 15 metastatic pure sRCC patients. No objective response was observed. Median TTP was 6.6 months, and six patients died from progressive disease before having access to the planned sorafenib second-line therapy [58]. The Eastern Cooperative Oncology Group (ECOG) performed a multicenter phase 2 study of doxorubicin-gemcitabine chemotherapy regimen in 39 patients with locally advanced or metastatic sRCC. Six (16%) patients achieved an objective response (five partial and one complete responses), and ten (26%) had a stable disease. The median OS was 8.8 months, and the median PFS was 3.5 months. The patient with a complete response and two of the five patients with partial response had more than 75% sarcomatoid differentiation. These patients had a prolonged PFS and OS compared to non-responders. The authors concluded that this

Table 9.2 Trials of cytokines or chemotherapy in sRCC

	Type of study	N	ccRCC subtype	Poor prognosis group (MSKCC or IMDC)	Treatment	Overall response rate	PFS$/TTP£/DFS€ (months)	OS (months)	Comparison with non-sRCC
Sella et al. [49]	Retrospective	44 (25 with metastatic disease)	NA	NA	Systemic treatment in 31 patients (chemotherapy, hormones, interferon)	6%a (2 CR with doxorubicin-containing regimen; no response with other treatments)	NA	13a	No
Culine et al. [50]	Retrospective	14 (with metastatic disease or recurrence)	NA	NA	IFNa: 4 Chemotherapy: 10 (8 with doxorubicin)	33%	NA	9 (prolonged survival >20 m for responding patients)	No
Wu et al. [51]	Retrospective	80 • 63 ccRCC • 10 cc sRCC • 7 pure sRCC	91%	NA	Cytokines (IL2 and IFNa)	Pure sRCC: 0	NA	Pure sRCC: 13.8	Yes Worse outcome for pure sRCC patients

Cangiano et al. [52]	Retrospective	31 (26 with metastasis)	NA	NA	24 patients: IL2 (alone or in combination with TILs and INFa), dendritic cell vaccine	21%[a]	NA	6.5 for all cohort	No
Escudier et al. [57]	Phase 2 prospective	23	NA	NA	Doxorubicin-ifosfamide	0	2.2[£]	3.9	No
Mian et al. [32]	Retrospective	108 (83 with metastasis)	82%	NA	86 patients: cytokines (IFNa, IL2) and/or chemotherapy	>30%	NA	9 for all cohort	No
Nanus et al. [53]	Retrospective	18 (10 sRCC)	NA	NA	Doxorubicin-gemcitabine	39%	NA	NA	No
Kwak et al. [54]	Retrospective	252 • 42 sRCC: (32 received cytokines; 10 did not receive cytokines) • 144 non-SRCC (93 received cytokines; 51 did not receive cytokines)	79% for sRCC	NA	IFNa alone or in combination with IL2 and 5FU	NA	3.2[a§] (9[a] for non-sRCC)	10 (22 for non-sRCC)	Yes Worse outcome for sRCC patients

(continued)

Table 9.2 (continued)

	Type of study	N	ccRCC subtype	Poor prognosis group (MSKCC or IMDC)	Treatment	Overall response rate	PFS§/TTP£/DFS€ (months)	OS (months)	Comparison with non-sRCC
Staehler et al. [58]	Phase 2 prospective	15	0 (pure sRCC)	0	Doxorubicin-gemcitabine (n = 15) Sorafenib at progression (n = 9)	Doxo-gem: 0 Sorafenib: 11%	Doxo-gem: 6.6£ Sorafenib: 10.9£	Sorafenib: 36.4	No
Jonasch et al. [61]	Phase 2 prospective	28 (10 sRCC)	61%	39%	Gemcitabine-capecitabine-bevacizumab	NA	5.9§ (3.9 for sRCC)	10.4 (9 for sRCC)	Yes Similar outcome
Dutcher et al. [55]	Retrospective	18	NA	NA	Doxorubicin-gemcitabine	39%	NA	NA Prolonged survival (>72 months) for 2 patients with CR	No
Roubaud et al. [56]	Retrospective	29 • 23 rapidly progressive non-sRCC • 6 sRCC	69% • 3 sRCC • 17 non-sRCC	NA	Doxorubicin-gemcitabine	7% (no response in sRCC)	3.7€	4.8	No
Haas et al. [59]	Phase 2 prospective (ECOG 8802)	39	74%	NA	Doxorubicin-gemcitabine	16%	3.5§	8.8	No

| Michaelson et al. [60] | Phase 2 prospective | 39 | 62% | 44% | Sunitinib–gemcitabine | 26% | 5$^£$ | 10 | No (but similar outcome to that of 33 poor-risk RC) |

ccRCC clear-cell renal cell carcinoma, *IMDC*, International Metastatic RCC Database Consortium, *MSKCC* Memorial Sloan Kettering Cancer Center, *PFS* progression-free survival, *TTP* time to progression, *DFS* disease-free survival, *OS* overall survival, *NA* not available, *CR* complete response, *IFNα* interferon alpha, *IL2* interleukin-2, *TILs* tumor-infiltrating lymphocytes

[a]For treated patients

chemotherapy combination, inactive in patients with mostly ccRCC, demonstrated interesting activity in patients with sRCC [59].

Michaelson et al. recently reported a phase 2 trial of gemcitabine associated with the targeted therapy sunitinib and in patients with sarcomatoid ($n = 39$) and/or poor-risk ($n = 33$) metastatic RCC. The overall response rate was 26% for patients with sRCC and 24% for patients with poor-risk RCC. The median TTP and OS for patients with sRCC were 5 and 10 months, respectively, quite similar with that of poor-risk patients (5.5 and 15 months) [60]. These results suggest that antiangio-genic therapy and cytotoxic chemotherapy are an active and well-tolerated combi-nation for patients with aggressive RCC, which may be more efficient than either therapy alone.

Jonasch et al. reported the results of a different association of chemotherapy (gem-citabine–capecitabine) and the targeted therapy bevacizumab, showing similar activ-ity in ten sRCC, with a median PFS of 3.9 months and median OS of 9 months [61].

Targeted Therapy

The large prospective randomized pivotal phase 3 clinical trials that had demon-strated a survival benefit of VEGFR- [62–65] or mTOR-targeted therapies [66, 67] in ccRCC did not describe either the specific outcome of patients with sarcomatoid differentiation.

Only data in limited cohorts, mostly retrospective, are available [2, 21, 25, 27, 34, 68–70]. These data are shown in Table 9.3.

There were only two small cohort phase 2 prospective studies that reported the outcome of sRCC patients treated with a sunitinib–gemcitabine combination [60] or with sorafenib after chemotherapy failure [58]. All the remaining studies were retrospective.

Targeted therapy was the only treatment assessed in seven studies, whereas the two remaining studies included patients also treated with chemotherapy or cytokines.

Targeted therapy was mostly given in the first-line setting, while a minority of patients had received previous treatment, including cytokines (interferon alpha and interleukin-2) in most cases.

All studies but one explored the role of VEGF-TT (sunitinib, sorafenib, pazo-panib, axitinib, and bevacizumab). Beuselinck et al. observed no objective response for the 11 patients with PSC $\geq$25% [34], while Park et al. reported the highest response rate with 45.8% of partial response in patients treated with VEGFR-TKIs [27]. No complete response was noted. Kunene et al. found that objective responses were observed only among the patients with a good performance status of 0 or 1 [70].

In the IMDC cohort, reported by Kyriakopoulos et al., the patients with sRCC ($n = 230$) had a worse tumor response than patients with non-sRCC ($n = 2056$), with a higher probability of primary refractory disease with first-line treatment (43% vs 21%, $p = $ <0.0001). In terms of subsequent treatment on disease progression, patients with sRCC were less likely to have a second- (37% vs 45%, $p = 0.0172$) and a third-line therapy (7% vs 16%, $p = 0.0004$) compared to non-sRCC patients [21].

Table 9.3 Trials of systemic targeted therapies in sRCC

	Type of study	N	ccRv CC subtype	Poor prognosis group (MSKCC* or IMDC&)	Treatment	First-line treatment	Overall response rate	PFS$/TTP£, median (months)	OS, Median (months)	Comparison with non-sRCC
Michaelson et al. [60]	Phase 2 prospective	39	62%	44%*	Sunitinib–gemcitabine	92%	26%	5£	10	No (but similar outcome to that of 33 poor-risk RCC)
Golshayan et al. [68]	Retrospective	43	77%	12%&	VEGF-TT (sunitinib, sorafenib, bevacizumab)	66%	19%	5.3$	11.8	No
Staehler et al. [58]	Phase 2 prospective	15	0 (pure sRCC)	0	Doxorubicin-gemcitabine (n = 15) Sorafenib at progression (n = 9)	Doxo-gem: 100%	Doxo-gem: 0 Sorafenib: 11%	Doxo-gem: 6.6£ Sorafenib: 10.9£	Sorafenib: 36.4	No
Molina et al. [25]	Retrospective	63	75%	5%*	VEGF-TT (alone or in combination): 51% Cytokine: 32% Other: 17%	100%	8%	3$	10	No

(continued)

Table 9.3 (continued)

	Type of study	N	ccRv CC subtype	Poor prognosis group (MSKCC* or IMDC&)	Treatment	First-line treatment	Overall response rate	PFS$/TTP£, median (months)	OS, Median (months)	Comparison with non-sRCC
Pal et al. [69]	Retrospective	21	62%	24%*/&	VEGF-TT (sunitinib, sorafenib): 57% Cytokine: 33% Chemotherapy: 10%	100%	NA	NA	18	No
Park et al. [27]	Retrospective	83	NA	NA	VEGF-TT (sunitinib, sorafenib, pazopanib)	83%	45.8%	12$	35	No
Beuselinck et al. [34]	Retrospective	117 • No PSC: 82 • PSC 1–24%: 24 • PSC ≥25%: 11	NA	38% for all cohort (82% if PCS ≥25%)	VEGF-TT (sunitinib, sorafenib, pazopanib)	NA	According to PSC: • <25%: 50% • ≥25%: 0	According to PSC: • <25%: 12$ • ≥25%: 3$	According to PSC: • <25%: 22 • ≥25%: 6	Yes (no statistical difference between non-sRCC and sRCC, but has statistical significance when compared <25% and ≥25%PSC on all cohort)
Kunene et al. [70]	Retrospective	23	78%	48%&	Sunitinib	79%	30%	5.7$	15.7	No

| Voss et al. [2] | Retrospective | 85 rapalog-treated patients: • 27% ccRCC with sarcomatoid features • 73% non ccRCC | 27% (all sRCC) | 17%* | For all cohort: Everolimus (30%) Temsirolimus (70%) | For all cohort: 35% | 7% (13% in sRCC) | 2.9§ (3.5 for sRCC) | 8.7 (8.2 for sRCC) | Yes Comparison with non ccRCC without sarcomatoid features. Poor outcome for both subgroups |
| Kyriakopoulos et al. [21] | Retrospective | 2208 • 230 with sRCC • 2056 with non-sRCC | • sRCC: 87% • n-sRCC: 88% | • sRCC: 40% • non-sRCC: 24% | VEGF-TT: >94% (>70% sunitinib) | 100% | • sRCC: 20% • non-sRCC: 26% | • sRCC: 4.5§ • non-sRCC: 7.8 | • sRCC: 10.4 • non-sRCC: 22.5 | Yes Patients with sRCC had a worse clinical outcome with targeted therapy |

*MSKCC and & to IMDC
§PFS and £ to TTP

ccRCC clear-cell renal cell carcinoma, IMDC International Metastatic RCC Database Consortium, MSKCC Memorial Sloan Kettering Cancer Center, PFS progression-free survival, TTP time to progression, OS overall survival, VEGF-TT vascular endothelial growth factor-targeted therapy, NA not available, PSC percentage of sarcomatoid component

Only one study focused on mTOR inhibitors. Voss et al. reported the outcome of ccRCC with sarcomatoid features (cc sRCC) and non-ccRCC treated with temsirolimus or everolimus, mostly in second- and third-line setting [2]. The authors reported that a subset of cc sRCC patients benefited from mTOR inhibitors, but most had poor outcome, as non-ccRCC patients.

Numakura et al. published a case report of a successful 19-month maintenance therapy with temsirolimus after two cycles of doxorubicin–gemcitabine chemotherapy in a 63-year-old patient with metastatic sRCC. However, no other report has confirmed these findings [71].

Immunotherapy: Immune Checkpoint Inhibitors

In 2015, Geynisman et al. described a case report of a 34-year-old man with a metastatic papillary RCC with sarcomatoid and rhabdoid features who had rapidly progressed after three lines of treatment including carboplatin–gemcitabine, sunitinib, and sunitinib–gemcitabine. The anti-programmed cell death protein-1 (PD-1) antibody nivolumab was introduced 6 months after the initial diagnosis and led to a dramatic clinical improvement, associated with an objective response on magnetic resonance and computed tomography imaging [72].

SRCC subgroup has not been described in the CheckMate025 phase 3 trial with nivolumab. However, Atezolizumab, an anti-PD-L1 antibody, has shown promising activity in the subgroup of 18 sRCC and/or Fuhrman 4 patients in a phase 1 study, with a median OS of 26.2 months, similar to that of the entire 62 patient cohorts (28.9 months) [73].

Translational research on molecular classification of ccRCC by Beuselinck et al. showed that the ccrcc4 subtype demonstrated specific features at the pathologic level with frequent sarcomatoid differentiation and inflammation [74]. Accordingly, pathway analysis of transcriptome profiles identified an overexpression of genes related to immune response, chemotaxis, and apoptosis, suggesting that this subtype could be particularly responsive to immune checkpoint inhibitors. A prospective biomarker-driven phase 2 study with nivolumab and ipilimumab or VEGFR-TKI, based on this molecular classification in naïve metastatic RCC, is ongoing to confirm these results (NCT02960906).

Conclusion

SRCC is a rare entity arising from any of the conventional histologic subtypes of RCC. Sarcomatoid differentiation is related to a poor prognosis in both localized and metastatic diseases, independently of the percentage of sarcomatoid component. For localized disease, surgery remains the standard of care, but adjuvant trial participation should be considered because of the high-risk for recurrence. In the metastatic setting, there may be a role for combination between chemotherapy and antiangiogenic therapy, even if survival is most often short. Immune checkpoint inhibitors seem to have a promising activity and should be specifically assessed. In parallel, better molecular and genetic characterization of sRCC will allow a better comprehension of this entity and the development of specific therapies.

References

1. Moch H, Humphrey P, Ulbright T, Reuter V. WHO classification of tumours of the urinary system and male genital organs. WHO/IARC classification of tumours, vol. 8. 4th ed; 2016.
2. Voss MH, Bastos DA, Karlo CA, Ajeti A, Hakimi AA, Feldman DR, et al. Treatment outcome with mTOR inhibitors for metastatic renal cell carcinoma with nonclear and sarcomatoid histologies. Ann Oncol. 2014;25(3):663–8.
3. de Peralta-Venturina M, Moch H, Amin M, Tamboli P, Hailemariam S, Mihatsch M, et al. Sarcomatoid differentiation in renal cell carcinoma: a study of 101 cases. Am J Surg Pathol. 2001;25(3):275–84.
4. Weisel W, Dockerty M, Priestley J. Sarcoma of the kidney. J Urol. 1943;50:564–73.
5. Farrow GM, Harrison EG, Utz DC, ReMine WH. Sarcomas and sarcomatoid and mixed malignant tumors of the kidney in adults. I. Cancer. 1968;22(3):545–50.
6. Bertoni F, Ferri C, Benati A, Bacchini P, Corrado F. Sarcomatoid carcinoma of the kidney. J Urol. 1987;137(1):25–8.
7. Störkel S, Eble JN, Adlakha K, Amin M, Blute ML, Bostwick DG, et al. Classification of renal cell carcinoma: Workgroup No. 1. Union Internationale Contre le Cancer (UICC) and the American Joint Committee on Cancer (AJCC). Cancer. 1997;80(5):987–9.
8. Lopez-Beltran A, Scarpelli M, Montironi R, Kirkali Z. 2004 WHO classification of the renal tumors of the adults. Eur Urol. 2006;49(5):798–805.
9. Delahunt B. Sarcomatoid renal carcinoma: the final common dedifferentiation pathway of renal epithelial malignancies. Pathology. 1999;31(3):185–90.
10. Boström AK, Möller C, Nilsson E, Elfving P, Axelson H, Johansson ME. Sarcomatoid conversion of clear cell renal cell carcinoma in relation to epithelial-to-mesenchymal transition. Hum Pathol. 2012;43(5):708–19.
11. Ro JY, Ayala AG, Sella A, Samuels ML, Swanson DA. Sarcomatoid renal cell carcinoma: clinicopathologic. A study of 42 cases. Cancer. 1987;59(3):516–26.
12. Delahunt B, Cheville JC, Martignoni G, Humphrey PA, Magi-Galluzzi C, McKenney J, et al. The International Society of Urological Pathology (ISUP) grading system for renal cell carcinoma and other prognostic parameters. Am J Surg Pathol. 2013;37(10):1490–504.
13. Sircar K, Yoo SY, Majewski T, Wani K, Patel LR, Voicu H, et al. Biphasic components of sarcomatoid clear cell renal cell carcinomas are molecularly similar to each other, but distinct from, non-sarcomatoid renal carcinomas. J Pathol Clin Res. 2015;1(4):212–24.
14. Cheville JC, Lohse CM, Zincke H, Weaver AL, Blute ML. Comparisons of outcome and prognostic features among histologic subtypes of renal cell carcinoma. Am J Surg Pathol. 2003;27(5):612–24.
15. Tickoo SK, Alden D, Olgac S, Fine SW, Russo P, Kondagunta GV, et al. Immunohistochemical expression of hypoxia inducible factor-1alpha and its downstream molecules in sarcomatoid renal cell carcinoma. J Urol. 2007;177(4):1258–63.
16. Conant JL, Peng Z, Evans MF, Naud S, Cooper K. Sarcomatoid renal cell carcinoma is an example of epithelial–mesenchymal transition. J Clin Pathol. 2011;64(12):1088–92.
17. Bi M, Zhao S, Said JW, Merino MJ, Adeniran AJ, Xie Z, et al. Genomic characterization of sarcomatoid transformation in clear cell renal cell carcinoma. Proc Natl Acad Sci U S A. 2016;113(8):2170–5.
18. Ito T, Pei J, Dulaimi E, Menges C, Abbosh PH, Smaldone MC, et al. Genomic copy number alterations in renal cell carcinoma with sarcomatoid features. J Urol. 2016;195(4 Pt 1):852–8.
19. Malouf GG, Ali SM, Wang K, Balasubramanian S, Ross JS, Miller VA, et al. Genomic characterization of renal cell carcinoma with sarcomatoid dedifferentiation pinpoints recurrent genomic alterations. Eur Urol. 2016;70(2):348–57.
20. Kim T, Zargar-Shoshtari K, Dhillon J, Lin HY, Yue B, Fishman M, et al. Using percentage of sarcomatoid differentiation as a prognostic factor in renal cell carcinoma. Clin Genitourin Cancer. 2015;13(3):225–30.

21. Kyriakopoulos CE, Chittoria N, Choueiri TK, Kroeger N, Lee JL, Srinivas S, et al. Outcome of patients with metastatic sarcomatoid renal cell carcinoma: results from the International Metastatic Renal Cell Carcinoma Database Consortium. Clin Genitourin Cancer. 2015;13(2):e79–85.

22. Pamela A, Arnoux V, Long JA, Rambeaud JJ, Lechevallier E. Sarcomatoid renal cell carcinoma: follow-up of a series of 23 patients. Prog Urol. 2014;24(5):301–6.

23. Cheville JC, Lohse CM, Zincke H, Weaver AL, Leibovich BC, Frank I, et al. Sarcomatoid renal cell carcinoma: an examination of underlying histologic subtype and an analysis of associations with patient outcome. Am J Surg Pathol. 2004;28(4):435–41.

24. Vera-Badillo FE, Templeton AJ, Duran I, Ocana A, de Gouveia P, Aneja P, et al. Systemic therapy for non-clear cell renal cell carcinomas: a systematic review and meta-analysis. Eur Urol. 2015;67(4):740–9.

25. Molina AM, Tickoo SK, Ishill N, Trinos MJ, Schwartz LH, Patil S, et al. Sarcomatoid-variant renal cell carcinoma: treatment outcome and survival in advanced disease. Am J Clin Oncol. 2011;34(5):454–9.

26. Nguyen DP, Vilaseca A, Vertosick EA, Corradi RB, Touijer KA, Benfante NE, et al. Histologic subtype impacts cancer-specific survival in patients with sarcomatoid-variant renal cell carcinoma treated surgically. World J Urol. 2016;34(4):539–44.

27. Park JY, Lee JL, Baek S, Eo SH, Go H, Ro JY, et al. Sarcomatoid features, necrosis, and grade are prognostic factors in metastatic clear cell renal cell carcinoma with vascular endothelial growth factor-targeted therapy. Hum Pathol. 2014;45(7):1437–44.

28. Brookman-May S, May M, Shariat SF, Zigeuner R, Chromecki T, Cindolo L, et al. Prognostic effect of sarcomatoid dedifferentiation in patients with surgically treated renal cell carcinoma: a matched-pair analysis. Clin Genitourin Cancer. 2013;11(4):465–70.

29. Shuch B, Bratslavsky G, Linehan WM, Srinivasan R. Sarcomatoid renal cell carcinoma: a comprehensive review of the biology and current treatment strategies. Oncologist. 2012;17(1):46–54.

30. Merrill MM, Wood CG, Tannir NM, Slack RS, Babaian KN, Jonasch E, et al. Clinically non-metastatic renal cell carcinoma with sarcomatoid dedifferentiation: natural history and outcomes after surgical resection with curative intent. Urol Oncol. 2015;33(4):166.e21–9.

31. Adibi M, Thomas AZ, Borregales LD, Merrill MM, Slack RS, Chen HC, et al. Percentage of sarcomatoid component as a prognostic indicator for survival in renal cell carcinoma with sarcomatoid dedifferentiation. Urol Oncol. 2015;33(10):427.e17–23.

32. Mian BM, Bhadkamkar N, Slaton JW, Pisters PW, Daliani D, Swanson DA, et al. Prognostic factors and survival of patients with sarcomatoid renal cell carcinoma. J Urol. 2002;167(1):65–70.

33. Shuch B, Bratslavsky G, Shih J, Vourganti S, Finley D, Castor B, et al. Impact of pathological tumour characteristics in patients with sarcomatoid renal cell carcinoma. BJU Int. 2012;109(11):1600–6.

34. Beuselinck B, Lerut E, Wolter P, Dumez H, Berkers J, Van Poppel H, et al. Sarcomatoid dedifferentiation in metastatic clear cell renal cell carcinoma and outcome on treatment with anti-vascular endothelial growth factor receptor tyrosine kinase inhibitors: a retrospective analysis. Clin Genitourin Cancer. 2014;12(5):e205–14.

35. Ljungberg B, Bensalah K, Canfield S, Dabestani S, Hofmann F, Hora M, et al. EAU guidelines on renal cell carcinoma: 2014 update. Eur Urol. 2015;67(5):913–24.

36. Zhang BY, Thompson RH, Lohse CM, Leibovich BC, Boorjian SA, Cheville JC, et al. A novel prognostic model for patients with sarcomatoid renal cell carcinoma. BJU Int. 2015;115(3):405–11.

37. Park DJ, Stoehlmacher J, Zhang W, Tsao-Wei DD, Groshen S, Lenz HJ. A Xeroderma pigmentosum group D gene polymorphism predicts clinical outcome to platinum-based chemotherapy in patients with advanced colorectal cancer. Cancer Res. 2001;61(24):8654–8.

38. Haas NB, Manola J, Uzzo RG, Flaherty KT, Wood CG, Kane C, et al. Adjuvant sunitinib or sorafenib for high-risk, non-metastatic renal-cell carcinoma (ECOG-ACRIN E2805): a double-blind, placebo-controlled, randomised, phase 3 trial. Lancet. 2016;387(10032):2008–16.

39. Ravaud A, Motzer RJ, Pandha HS, George DJ, Pantuck AJ, Patel A, et al. Adjuvant sunitinib in high-risk renal-cell carcinoma after nephrectomy. N Engl J Med. 2016;375(23):2246–54.
40. Eminaga O, Akbarov I, Wille S, Engelmann U. Does postoperative radiation therapy impact survival in non-metastatic sarcomatoid renal cell carcinoma? A SEER-based study. Int Urol Nephrol. 2015;47(10):1653–63.
41. Mickisch GH, Garin A, van Poppel H, de Prijck L, Sylvester R, Group EOfRaToCEG. Radical nephrectomy plus interferon-alfa-based immunotherapy compared with interferon alfa alone in metastatic renal-cell carcinoma: a randomised trial. Lancet. 2001;358(9286):966–70.
42. Flanigan RC, Salmon SE, Blumenstein BA, Bearman SI, Roy V, McGrath PC, et al. Nephrectomy followed by interferon alfa-2b compared with interferon alfa-2b alone for metastatic renal-cell cancer. N Engl J Med. 2001;345(23):1655–9.
43. Heng DY, Wells JC, Rini BI, Beuselinck B, Lee JL, Knox JJ, et al. Cytoreductive nephrectomy in patients with synchronous metastases from renal cell carcinoma: results from the International Metastatic Renal Cell Carcinoma Database Consortium. Eur Urol. 2014;66(4):704–10.
44. Shuch B, Said J, La Rochelle JC, Zhou Y, Li G, Klatte T, et al. Cytoreductive nephrectomy for kidney cancer with sarcomatoid histology-is up-front resection indicated and, if not, is it avoidable? J Urol. 2009;182(5):2164–71.
45. Thomas AZ, Adibi M, Slack RS, Borregales LD, Merrill MM, Tamboli P, et al. The Role of metastasectomy in patients with renal cell carcinoma with sarcomatoid dedifferentiation: a matched controlled analysis. J Urol. 2016;196(3):678–84.
46. Escudier B, Bellmunt J, Négrier S, Bajetta E, Melichar B, Bracarda S, et al. Phase III trial of bevacizumab plus interferon alfa-2a in patients with metastatic renal cell carcinoma (AVOREN): final analysis of overall survival. J Clin Oncol. 2010;28(13):2144–50.
47. Rini BI, Halabi S, Rosenberg JE, Stadler WM, Vaena DA, Archer L, et al. Phase III trial of bevacizumab plus interferon alfa versus interferon alfa monotherapy in patients with metastatic renal cell carcinoma: final results of CALGB 90206. J Clin Oncol. 2010;28(13):2137–43.
48. Negrier S, Escudier B, Lasset C, Douillard JY, Savary J, Chevreau C, et al. Recombinant human interleukin-2, recombinant human interferon alfa-2a, or both in metastatic renal-cell carcinoma. Groupe Français d'Immunothérapie. N Engl J Med. 1998;338(18):1272–8.
49. Sella A, Logothetis CJ, Ro JY, Swanson DA, Samuels ML. Sarcomatoid renal cell carcinoma. A treatable entity. Cancer. 1987;60(6):1313–8.
50. Culine S, Bekradda M, Terrier-Lacombe MJ, Droz JP. Treatment of sarcomatoid renal cell carcinoma: is there a role for chemotherapy? Eur Urol. 1995;27(2):138–41.
51. Wu J, Caliendo G, Hu XP, Dutcher JP. Impact of histology on the treatment outcome of metastatic or recurrent renal cell carcinoma. Med Oncol. 1998;15(1):44–9.
52. Cangiano T, Liao J, Naitoh J, Dorey F, Figlin R, Belldegrun A. Sarcomatoid renal cell carcinoma: biologic behavior, prognosis, and response to combined surgical resection and immunotherapy. J Clin Oncol. 1999;17(2):523–8.
53. Nanus DM, Garino A, Milowsky MI, Larkin M, Dutcher JP. Active chemotherapy for sarcomatoid and rapidly progressing renal cell carcinoma. Cancer. 2004;101(7):1545–51.
54. Kwak C, Park YH, Jeong CW, Jeong H, Lee SE, Moon KC, et al. Sarcomatoid differentiation as a prognostic factor for immunotherapy in metastatic renal cell carcinoma. J Surg Oncol. 2007;95(4):317–23.
55. Dutcher JP, Nanus D. Long-term survival of patients with sarcomatoid renal cell cancer treated with chemotherapy. Med Oncol. 2011;28(4):1530–3.
56. Roubaud G, Gross-Goupil M, Wallerand H, de Clermont H, Dilhuydy MS, Ravaud A. Combination of gemcitabine and doxorubicin in rapidly progressive metastatic renal cell carcinoma and/or sarcomatoid renal cell carcinoma. Oncology. 2011;80(3–4):214–8.
57. Escudier B, Droz JP, Rolland F, Terrier-Lacombe MJ, Gravis G, Beuzeboc P, et al. Doxorubicin and ifosfamide in patients with metastatic sarcomatoid renal cell carcinoma: a phase II study of the Genitourinary Group of the French Federation of Cancer Centers. J Urol. 2002;168(3):959–61.

58. Staehler M, Haseke N, Roosen A, Stadler T, Bader M, Siebels M, et al. Sorafenib after combination therapy with gemcitabine plus doxorubicine in patients with sarcomatoid renal cell carcinoma: a prospective evaluation. Eur J Med Res. 2010;15:287–91.
59. Haas NB, Lin X, Manola J, Pins M, Liu G, McDermott D, et al. A phase II trial of doxorubicin and gemcitabine in renal cell carcinoma with sarcomatoid features: ECOG 8802. Med Oncol. 2012;29(2):761–7.
60. Michaelson MD, McKay RR, Werner L, Atkins MB, Van Allen EM, Olivier KM, et al. Phase 2 trial of sunitinib and gemcitabine in patients with sarcomatoid and/or poor-risk metastatic renal cell carcinoma. Cancer. 2015;121(19):3435–43.
61. Jonasch E, Lal LS, Atkinson BJ, Byfield SD, Miller LA, Pagliaro LC, et al. Treatment of metastatic renal carcinoma patients with the combination of gemcitabine, capecitabine and bevacizumab at a tertiary cancer centre. BJU Int. 2011;107(5):741–7.
62. Motzer RJ, Hutson TE, Tomczak P, Michaelson MD, Bukowski RM, Rixe O, et al. Sunitinib versus interferon alfa in metastatic renal-cell carcinoma. N Engl J Med. 2007;356(2):115–24.
63. Motzer RJ, McCann L, Deen K. Pazopanib versus sunitinib in renal cancer. N Engl J Med. 2013;369(20):1970.
64. Sternberg CN, Davis ID, Mardiak J, Szczylik C, Lee E, Wagstaff J, et al. Pazopanib in locally advanced or metastatic renal cell carcinoma: results of a randomized phase III trial. J Clin Oncol. 2010;28(6):1061–8.
65. Rini BI, Escudier B, Tomczak P, Kaprin A, Szczylik C, Hutson TE, et al. Comparative effectiveness of axitinib versus sorafenib in advanced renal cell carcinoma (AXIS): a randomised phase 3 trial. Lancet. 2011;378(9807):1931–9.
66. Motzer RJ, Escudier B, Oudard S, Hutson TE, Porta C, Bracarda S, et al. Efficacy of everolimus in advanced renal cell carcinoma: a double-blind, randomised, placebo-controlled phase III trial. Lancet. 2008;372(9637):449–56.
67. Hudes G, Carducci M, Tomczak P, Dutcher J, Figlin R, Kapoor A, et al. Temsirolimus, interferon alfa, or both for advanced renal-cell carcinoma. N Engl J Med. 2007;356(22):2271–81.
68. Golshayan AR, George S, Heng DY, Elson P, Wood LS, Mekhail TM, et al. Metastatic sarcomatoid renal cell carcinoma treated with vascular endothelial growth factor-targeted therapy. J Clin Oncol. 2009;27(2):235–41.
69. Pal SK, Jones JO, Carmichael C, Saikia J, Hsu J, Liu X, et al. Clinical outcome in patients receiving systemic therapy for metastatic sarcomatoid renal cell carcinoma: a retrospective analysis. Urol Oncol. 2013;31(8):1826–31.
70. Kunene V, Miscoria M, Pirrie S, Islam MR, Afshar M, Porfiri E. Sarcomatoid renal cell carcinoma: clinical outcome and survival after treatment with sunitinib. Clin Genitourin Cancer. 2014;12(4):251–5.
71. Numakura K, Tsuchiya N, Akihama S, Inoue T, Narita S, Huang M, et al. Successful mammalian target of rapamycin inhibitor maintenance therapy following induction chemotherapy with gemcitabine and doxorubicin for metastatic sarcomatoid renal cell carcinoma. Oncol Lett. 2014;8(1):464–6.
72. Geynisman DM. Anti-programmed cell death protein 1 (pd-1) antibody nivolumab leads to a dramatic and rapid response in papillary renal cell carcinoma with sarcomatoid and rhabdoid features. Eur Urol. 2015;68(5):912–4.
73. McDermott DF, Sosman JA, Sznol M, Massard C, Gordon MS, Hamid O, et al. Atezolizumab, an anti-programmed death-ligand 1 antibody, in metastatic renal cell carcinoma: long-term safety, clinical activity, and immune correlates from a phase ia study. J Clin Oncol. 2016;34(8):833–42.
74. Beuselinck B, Job S, Becht E, Karadimou A, Verkarre V, Couchy G, et al. Molecular subtypes of clear cell renal cell carcinoma are associated with sunitinib response in the metastatic setting. Clin Cancer Res. 2015;21(6):1329–39.